PRAISE FOR *THE ORDER OF THINGS*

"Sarah Gormley's debut memoir is much more than the story of one woman who confronted her unhappiness and marched toward a better life. It is also a beautifully written testament to doing the hard work of changing your circumstances and opening your heart to a more meaningful life filled with hope and love. This story will resonate with any woman who has spent time chasing gold stars only to end up exhausted, lonely, and unfulfilled. Gormley's a towering talent and a writer to watch!"

—Christie Tate, *New York Times* bestselling
author of *Group* and *B.F.F.*

"In *The Order of Things*, Sarah Gormley invites us into the depths of her life experiences, from the triumphs of her career to the shadows of self-doubt, and ultimately to powerful transformation. With honesty and humor, she offers profound insights into the process of self-discovery and the beautiful complexity of real change. Gormley's story is truly one about self-hope and the endless possibilities that come with embracing one's true self."

—Fran Hauser, bestselling author, speaker, entrepreneur,
media executive, and women's champion

"I've been waiting for this book since I heard Sarah speak at DePauw University in 2019, where I instantly fell in love with her as she described leaving her high-powered job to care for her mother. Now, through her generous, beautiful book, I feel like she's my best friend.

The Order of Things is tender and sassy and real, like Sarah herself. I didn't want this book to end, so I just might read it again and again!"
—Meg Kissinger, award-winning journalist and author of *While You Were Out*

"In her poignant yet humor-laden debut, Gormley invites readers on an introspective journey through the tangled pathways of womanhood. With unflinching honesty and a generous sprinkle of wit, Gormley tackles the universal question that echoes in the minds of women everywhere: How did my life turn out this way?"
—Jo Piazza, national and international bestselling author of *The Sicilian Inheritance* and *We Are Not Like Them*

"Lots of books tell us what to do to change our lives, but very few actually *show* us what real change looks like. This book will make you laugh and cry at the same time, and you'll be astounded by Gormley's ability to write so beautifully about the messiness of life. Easy to read and impossible to put down, *The Order of Things* should be on your must-read list."
—Bonnie Wan, strategist, speaker, and author of *The Life Brief*

"When you know a person well, you can be in touch with their inner essence, their inner core—the most essential part of them. Sarah has a golden core."
—David, Sarah's Therapist

THE
ORDER
OF
THINGS

THE ORDER OF THINGS

A Memoir about Chasing Joy

SARAH GORMLEY

SALT CREEK PUBLISHING

Published by Salt Creek Publishing, Columbus, Ohio
www.sarahgormley.com
www.sarahgormleygallery.com

Cover art by Joey Monsoon

Design: Paul Barrett
Project management: Mari Kesselring and Emilie Sandoz-Voyer
Editorial production: Reshma Kooner

ISBN (hardcover): 979-8-9906425-0-8
ISBN (ebook): 979-8-9906425-1-5

Library of Congress Control Number is available.

First edition

For Mom

"DON'T HESITATE"

By Mary Oliver

If you suddenly and unexpectedly feel joy,
don't hesitate. Give in to it. There are plenty
of lives and whole towns destroyed or about
to be. We are not wise, and not very often
kind. And much can never be redeemed.
Still, life has some possibility left. Perhaps this
is its way of fighting back, that sometimes
something happens better than all the riches
or power in the world. It could be anything,
but very likely you notice it in the instant
when love begins. Anyway, that's often the
case. Anyway, whatever it is, don't be afraid
of its plenty. Joy is not made to be a crumb.

AUTHOR'S NOTE

New York City, 2001

I was twenty-nine years old and desperately wanted to figure out what was wrong with me.

I picked up my preordered copy of *The Noonday Demon: An Atlas of Depression* and read from the time I got home from work until three o'clock in the morning on the yellow sofa in my tiny apartment on the Upper East Side. I flipped ahead, scanning for a sentence or paragraph, something I could relate to in Andrew Solomon's story of emotional anguish. I was disappointed when I didn't see myself in his pages.

There were other books too; I hoped to find answers in Susanna Kaysen's *Girl, Interrupted* or Elizabeth Wurtzel's *Prozac Nation*, but my situation didn't seem to match up with theirs either. I felt let down when I couldn't find the answer I was searching for. I didn't feel the aches of sadness and despair that people suffering from depression experienced. I wasn't despondent or suicidal. I wasn't manic or a drug addict or any of the things I believed to be indicators of mental illness. In fact, if you had asked me, I would have told you how fortunate I was to have a loving family, a circle of wonderful friends, and an interesting career. I knew I was lucky. I could see and appreciate the splendid tapestry of the world around me, even at my worst.

And yet, I was mired in thick and unrelenting self-loathing that accompanied me through every step of my day. No matter what I accomplished externally—what I tracked as my ever-growing list of gold stars—I couldn't quell the voice that told me over and over that I was a failure, an absolute piece of shit who wasn't good enough. I couldn't remember a time I didn't feel this way. The pattern was so strong, I couldn't imagine who I would be without the constant companion of self-hatred.

Therapy seemed like another potential source for answers, so I found a therapist not far from my apartment. He wore tiny, wire-rimmed glasses that rested on the end of his nose, glasses that would be selected only by a man who wanted to appear intellectual. I was wearing a black-and-white silk wrap dress that I purchased from the clearance sale rack at Bergdorf's. This therapist looked at me and the dress when I entered his office, and—I'm not making this up—said, "You're thin and attractive. What could be bothering you?"

I sat there stunned and speechless. He kept asking me to explain why I felt so poorly about myself. I wanted to strangle him. If I knew why I was feeling this way, why the fuck would I need him, with his tiny glasses? I left that session feeling as if I had made a mistake going to see him, and the next week, I felt certain it was a mistake when he called me "Rebecca" after I sat down. I wondered if she was thin and attractive too. I didn't go back. I didn't try therapy again for eleven more years, and looking back, I can see that I wasn't yet ready to do the work. Instead, I continued to look for books that might have parallels to what I was experiencing.

I wanted a book to show me I wasn't alone, that somebody else had these feelings for as long as I had, but then somehow recovered. I wanted to read about a woman who appeared to have it all together but was suffering beneath the surface. I wanted to understand what she did to quiet the voice in her head and feel better.

I wanted to read something that would give me hope.

I wrote this book largely to understand what happened to me, but I also wrote this book for the younger version of me, the one on the yellow sofa looking for answers.

PROLOGUE

A LITTLE GIRL GETS OFF THE BUS

I can't wait to get home. I'm on the kindergarten bus on a late-spring Friday afternoon in Ohio. We go past the Okey Farm, the Terrill Farm, and then the old white houses and the small herds of cattle flicking their tails to keep the first of the summer flies away. I'm five years old, a freckled tomboy with short, dirty-blond hair, wearing my brother's hand-me-down Levi's and worn sneakers Mrs. Ferris double knotted before I left school. I'm wearing the green cotton shirt I wear almost every day because I like to chew on the white ties that hang down from the collar.

We turn left onto Clay Pike and cross the first of the two bridges that bookend our property, which is called Salt Creek Farm. I can't yet read, but I know from the way the words look on the envelopes I bring in from the mailbox that sometimes things are sent to 6535 Clay Pike, sometimes Rural Route 1, and sometimes just Salt Creek Farm. I wonder how my home can be called so many different things if it's all the same place.

I move up to the front seat behind Mr. Baker, the bus driver. He smells like detergent and chewing tobacco and wears a short-sleeve plaid button-down and a black watch on his right wrist. He pushes on the brake with his foot and reaches over to pull the crank to open the bus door that folds in on itself like an accordion. We're finally here.

"Let's see it, Sarah," he says, knowing what I'm about to do.

I jump down all three steps, which I've been working on all year. I can finally make it over the last two and land squarely on the dusty road, a few feet from our long gravel driveway. I turn to wave at Mr. Baker, who winks and gives me a thumbs-up before the yellow bus continues up the road past Salt Creek Baptist Church on the left, down the hill, across the second bridge, and around the big curve on the way up to the McLoughlins, our closest neighbors, who live a mile away.

I think about stopping to pick some daffodils from the large bed at the bottom of the driveway, but I don't have a paper towel and don't like the way the liquid oozes out of the bottom of the stems. Besides, I can't afford to waste any time. I start running—maybe half-skipping but faster than walking. I'm glad my shoes are double knotted because I've fallen so many times, and the edges of the gravel are sharp. I need to get to the house because Mom will be waiting for me. I've been looking forward to this moment all day, ever since I got on the bus that morning. Jane and Joe won't be home from school for another hour, so this time with her is all mine. Just Mom and me, the two of us.

She toasts onion bagels topped with Havarti under the broiler until the cheese bubbles down the sides. I climb into her lap, and we eat our bagels as we watch *Another World* together. I've been worried all week and have to ask, "Are Mac and Rachel really going to get a divorce?" which makes Mom laugh. After we finish our bagels, I lean onto her chest and feel the warmth of her body through the back of my green shirt. If I'm very quiet and still, I swear I can hear our hearts beating at the same time.

A WOMAN RETURNS TO THE FARM

I'm forty-five years old, and the farm still smells the same, like baby calves born earlier in the year and frost that has burned off the field from the November afternoon sun. The rhythm of our family changed when Dad died, but this place is still the only place I've called home. I want to sit at the bottom of the driveway for as long as I can. I want somebody to hit the pause button on me so that the beauty of this place might blanket the mess of my life, but I know Mom is waiting.

I don't know whether to turn right or left when I get to the top of the driveway.

My brother Joe will be over at the barn if I turn right, but I know that Mom will be at the house in the other direction. I rented a car rather than ask anyone to pick me up from the airport, and I wonder how being on that gravel driveway will feel this time. A line of grass grew up the middle the way Mom had always wanted, and the gravel seemed to behave for her, staying where it was supposed to be in two neat lanes.

As a little girl my feet toughened so much from our barefoot summer days that I could run on the sharp points of that chalky limestone with no shoes. My feet hold memories of the farm. I believe it became part of us, and in return we became part of it through a visceral connection with the land. *Symbiotic* is the word from ninth-grade biology—when two organisms form a mutually beneficial relationship, depending on each other to stay alive. I feel that way about the farm.

When I get to the top of the driveway, I see Joe standing outside the metal round barn with Camillus Musselman, a cousin of our neighbors and one of Joe's best friends. I haven't seen Camillus since the Fourth of July, but I know he's been spending more time at the farm because he's going through a tough divorce. The farm has always been a good place to get away. He's sparkly—always has been—and his eyes light up when he smiles. Camillus looks confused that I'm here on a nonholiday Sunday.

"Hey, Sarah . . . what are you doing at home? What's going on?"

"Oh, Mom has a few appointments that are probably nothing. I thought I'd go with her—no big deal. Back to San Francisco on Tuesday."

I try to be nonchalant even though I can hear my voice crack and feel my eyes start to well up. Camillus looks at me like he doesn't believe this is no big deal, and then he turns toward Joe, who gives him a look that says *Stop asking questions*. The three of us stop making eye contact. Camillus kicks at the gravel.

Joe gives me a hug and tells me Mom is over at the house, which I already know. I also know she hasn't left the house since the day before, when we found out she had tumors up and down her spine.

KNOWING VERSUS *KNOWING*

Mom opens the door and looks at me as I walk up the two steps of the breezeway Joe built to connect the garage to the house after Dad had slipped on some ice years before. She looks smaller than when I last saw her, two months before. She makes a face, her nose and lips rising up, the face you might make when you taste something bad, but in our family it is the this-isn't-good face.

I don't know what to say, so I yell as loud as I can:

"FUUUUUUUUUUUUUUUUUUUUUUCK!"

Mom smiles and steps toward me. She yells as loud as she can:

"FUUUUUUUUUUUUUUUUUUUUUUCK!"

We keep yelling at and with each other.

"FUUUUUUUUUUCK!"

"FUUUUUUCKITY FUUUUUUUUCK!"

"FUUUUUUUUCK!"

"FUUUUUCK!"

"FUUUUUCK!"

We don't laugh. The yelling helps us survive at least this moment, when we see each other and know what each of us knows. I hug her longer than normal and as tightly as I can, even though I am afraid I might feel the tumors through her sweater. I follow her into the front room, which is where she spends most of her time, sitting in Dad's chair by the window, where she can watch the birds at the feeder and see who might be coming up the driveway. We still call it "his" chair even though Dad died the year before, and we're still trying to adjust to his absence in our lives and in this house.

I let her see my tears.

"I'm so sorry, Mom. God, this sucks," I say. "I don't know what I'm supposed to say. How are you feeling right now?"

"Oh, Sarah," she says. "It does suck. I'm a little pissed off, to tell you the truth, but at least now I know why I've been feeling like shit for so long."

"Well, what if the ER guy made a mistake?" I ask. "I mean, we have to get more information at the appointment with your actual doctor tomorrow, right?" I am still in shock that an ER doctor told my sister that Mom had cancer the day before.

She looks at me for a moment, hesitating. "Honey, I know I'm really sick," she says. "I can feel it in my bones and also *in my bones*. I know."

I put my face in my hands, crying harder, but still nodding because I want her to know that I hear her. I take some deep breaths and smile, thinking how odd it is to be having this conversation with her, and yet how normal it feels. The setting is familiar, the sounds of our voices filling up the old house, the words themselves a comfort because we know what we sound like together.

"I need to tell you something," I say. "I've decided that whatever we find out, I'm coming home to be with you during your treatment."

I expect her to protest and tell me to stay in San Francisco. She knows that my big, important job at Adobe is in jeopardy. I assume she won't want me to do anything to make my situation worse.

"I'd really like for you to come home if you can," she says. "I feel better when you're here."

I nod and get up to go to the kitchen for a glass of water because I can feel an awful truth taking over my body. I don't want her to see the tears morphing into shoulder-heaving silent sobs. Yes, Mom told me she knew she was really sick, and yes, I heard her. But the moment she agreed to my coming home, something shifted. There is knowing in your brain, and there is *knowing* in your body. You feel it in your bones. *In your fucking bones.*

Standing there in front of the same sink that leaked slightly at the base of the faucet since I was a little girl, I realize I might be coming home to help her die.

FOUR DAYS BEFORE THAT DAY

1. I looked at the red canvas carry-on bag, the only suitcase I owned. Turns out I'm an incredibly light packer. After I joined Adobe in San Francisco, the bag went with me to France, Japan, Australia, New York, Vegas, and countless overnight trips to San Jose for meetings at the mother ship.
2. I loved and hated that red bag.
3. One of my bad cats, Howard Hughes, was lying on top of the bag. He knew I was leaving again, and I used a lint roller to remove his black hair before the car service came to pick me up. I was headed to San Francisco International Airport, so I could fly to New York, where I had meetings and was slated to talk about something or other at a conference created to support women in advertising.
4. I leaned my head back and prayed that the driver would stop asking me about where I was going and what I did and whether I liked living in Pacific Heights and if I could see the Golden Gate Bridge from the top of my building. I could see the bridge. But I didn't care.
5. Except I did care. I knew how lucky I was. I'd been reminding myself how lucky I was for as long as I could remember so that when the work stress and self-doubt

and self-loathing crept in, I could bring myself back with the knowledge I was lucky.

6. But also, I was tired.

7. Three weeks before, I was in Vegas for a big Adobe conference.

8. After that I met my DePauw girls for four days in Monterey for our forty-fifth birthday trip. I knew what love felt like when I was with them.

9. These girls knew about the situation at work, but they were accustomed to my stress because I'd been this way for almost twenty years.

10. Now the stress felt different. With my therapist's help, I realized that there's the real stress of work but also the more significant stress of not changing your life when you know it's time.

11. I thought I might get fired. I needed to quit. I interviewed at Google for another big job in big tech, which I knew would be another mistake, but I didn't know what else to do. I interviewed with a fashion startup, which felt like a bigger mistake because it was the same amount of stress without the same amount of money.

12. My job was not my life, but I couldn't figure out what my life was without my job.

13. I was worried about Mom. Over Labor Day weekend, I took her to a little ranch in Colorado. She had pain in her back, and she was having some stomach issues. She was exhausted all of the time. We thought it could be lingering grief from Dad dying the year before, but nobody knew for sure.

14. I said goodbye to her at the airport in Denver, where she flew back to Ohio and I flew back to San Francisco. I waited until she boarded before I let the tears come. She was one half of my parents, the only half left.

15. I got to New York, to some hotel, where I dialed into meetings from the room and worked on the slides for the next meeting until it was time to go to the conference.

16. Adobe was a sponsor, and I was introducing something or somebody important on the main stage.
17. I decided to stay for the weekend and visit my friends Mark and Kim because seeing them always made me feel okay about life.
18. They told me to hang in there, that it would get better, that I would figure something out. That I always did.
19. We were about to leave for dinner when my sister called from outside an emergency room in Ohio.
20. She told me that Mom had cancer up and down her spine.
21. I didn't understand what she said.
22. She repeated what she said—that scans showed nodules up and down Mom's spine.
23. I didn't understand how somebody in an emergency room, maybe not even a real fucking doctor, just told us that Mom had cancer.
24. Mark and Kim watched me try not to sob in their kitchen. The doors and windows were open, and I could feel the breeze. Things were still moving somehow. I was there, but I was not there.
25. I did not fly back to San Francisco the next day.
26. I packed my red canvas bag and flew home to Ohio.

FOUR DAYS AFTER THAT DAY

Usually, I simply tell people I *left* Adobe. Sometimes, I say Adobe *fired* me.

And other times, I go into a thorough explanation about how when you're at that level and things aren't working out, you enter into an agreement called a "mutual separation," which sounds just as absurd as the new term for breaking up, "conscious uncoupling," until you're actually one half of the mutually separated. The employee agrees that the situation isn't working and will leave without much fuss—the fuss being an expensive lawsuit and settlement the company wants to avoid—and in return for no fuss and a signed NDA, the company pays you some agreed-upon severance. Money helps make everyone feel a little bit better about a shitty situation.

The specific order of things is that Adobe fired me even though I was going to leave.

The broader order of things is that Adobe was just another big job with another big title I never should have taken in the first place.

You might want to hate Adobe for firing me rather than letting me take a leave of absence just days after I told them my mom likely was dying. I hated them for a while, but now I see things differently. We know things now that we didn't know back then.

A quick series of scenes in a movie would show our heroine climbing her way to better brands, bigger salaries, and meetings in boardrooms with this or that CEO. All of these things happened to make me *an executive* and *successful*. I did the work, and I hoped the sense of accomplishment would make me feel better about myself.

I'd started therapy, which slowly helped me understand my attachment to success, but Mom's cancer provided a shock of perspective on how badly I wanted my life to change. I decide to go home and, no matter what happened with her, take a full year off and live on the farm.

I put all of my possessions in storage and take home the things I think I might need for what I begin to call my "grown-up gap year." I pack boots, jeans, and cashmere sweaters for a trip I didn't yet know was going to become my life.

WHAT YOU NEED TO KNOW

I want to tell you a story.

I could tell you the full story of the little girl who got off the bus when she was five all the way to forty-five, filling in all of the years through the chapters. If I were funny and descriptive enough, using active dialogue and showing not telling, as writing teachers say, you might keep reading page after page, book after book. Hell, my haircuts alone could inspire a pretty large collection of essays. But that's not the story—at least not the story I want to tell you.

There was a little girl who grew up on a farm, and there was a woman who came back to that same farm when her mother's cancer returned.

I'm trying to figure out what happened to her.

I'm trying to figure out what happened to me.

If I can piece together the things that matter—the farm, my family, my mother—and make sense of the relationships between them, then that will help me better understand.

Most stories unfold like this: this thing happened and that thing happened and then this thing over there happened, too, by the way, and then you have a conclusion that makes sense. The end. Isn't that remarkable? But who decides what matters? How do we become who we are, and in what order? There's an order of time—chronology and calendars and what happened. But there's also the order of magnitude—what happened that made a difference, and how one moment matters more than four years. I'm learning that the order changes continuously, which makes it hard to tell a neat and tidy story. Who truly knows what things are causal versus merely correlated when it comes to our identities? What if the thing you think mattered most isn't what mattered at all?

DOCTOR'S APPOINTMENT

Joe comes in through the front door with the *Times Recorder* under his arm before he goes out to feed the mooing herd of Angus cattle, who run to the fence when they see his truck coming up the driveway. Joe and his wife, Christi, moved home from Nantucket after their son was born. They live in a cabin that Joe built, nestled down in the woods next to a ravine. The rustic cabin has a green tin roof that sings when it rains. He now takes care of the property and the cattle, as well as the remaining oil wells our family has owned for generations. Joe is talented and brilliant and the kind of guy who can do all of these things as if it's normal to be able to do all of these things. I hate thinking about the pain he's in worrying about Mom. He's in his farmer uniform: Carhartt jeans, rubber work boots, and an orange wool knit hat folded down on his head that makes him look vaguely gnomelike.

"Good morning," he says, making subtle eye contact with me to get a read on the mood in the room. I smile and nod, telling him we're okay without saying anything. He doesn't sit down. This isn't a let's-chat visit; it's a let's-check-in-to-see-how-we're-doing visit.

"Are you all set to take her to her appointment?" Joe asks when Mom is in the kitchen.

"Yes, all good. Jane offered to take the day off work, but I told her I'm here now, so I'm happy to go."

Jane also lives fairly close with her husband and their children. She's always wanted nothing but goodness in the world and for her family. I'm worried about Jane too—how Mom being sick will affect her. Somehow, we all made it through losing Dad, and we felt like a team, always with Mom at the center. Dad died just last year, and part of the gut punch of potentially losing Mom is the cruel timeline. Without Mom to ground us, how would we ever be a family again? How would we even know what to do? How does anyone do this? It feels impossible, but other people—more than anyone wants to believe—have to go through this all of the time.

Joe shuts the door behind him, and we watch as his truck heads over to the barns.

"What a nice boy. He takes such good care of me," Mom says. I can tell she is saying this more to herself than to me, and I understand that she's already started to take stock of her life. I watch her and see her processing what I am trying not to accept—that she might be coming to the end of her life.

**

Dr. Wegner looks to be about fifty, with silver hair, dark eyes that twinkle, and the demeanor of a man who might be an oncologist, or who might sell antique books.

He is quiet. His hands stay close to his body as he talks and makes eye contact. His eyes say *I know how hard this is* without saying anything aloud. I find his presence reassuring. I wonder how medical schools test for demeanor and whether students get bonus points for how they handle this type of conversation. He's reviewed the scans from the emergency room. He looks at Mom.

"Susan, unfortunately, I believe the tumors likely are cancerous, but

I'm reluctant to say anything more until they've done a second set of scans and the necessary blood work."

I refrain from asking him if he thinks it's okay that some kid—I have no idea how old or how degreed that person was, but I am choosing to hate *him* for telling my sister my mom has cancer on a Saturday visit to the ER for back pain—informed us prematurely.

"How long until we have results?" I ask, already wondering what we need to do next. I'm approaching Mom's cancer like a problem to be solved, the same way I've approached everything else in my life—as if there's a formula, as if my actions can help create order. In my mind, if I do A and B, then C should happen. There is no other way. Except I know that's not true. Dad died last year, and now here we are again, in a hospital room, waiting.

Dr. Wegner's face is kind. He smiles in a way that calms me, despite the fact we're sitting here talking about cancer. And even though I'm asking the questions, he directs his answers to Mom, and I like this about him. She's the patient; she matters most because we are talking about her life.

"We will get the results early next week. The blood work always takes longer than you might think, so I want to manage your expectations. I will call you once I've reviewed everything, and we can go from there. How does that sound?"

Mom smiles back at him, but it's her sarcastic smile.

"Well, it doesn't sound as good as going home and taking a nap."

Dr. Wegner stands up, and I notice how he touches Mom's shoulder when he leaves the room. Not a squeeze and not a pat—just a gentle touch that might seem too familiar coming from a stranger but from him it's a small gesture of kindness and knowing.

A few minutes later, a nurse comes in to draw blood. She has a bright pink manicure with tiny rhinestones on the tips, and I wonder how often she has to have her nails done. I wonder if her mother is healthy and about how many mother-and-daughter pairs she sees every day. I watch Mom's blood pool into the little glass vial and think about the week ahead—what we will do while we wait for a tablespoon of blood to tell us what's coming next.

PARKING LOT THERAPY

The next day, I work out at Schimmel's Gym, where Mom has gone for personal training sessions two times a week for the past ten years. I ask Bill, the owner and trainer, if it's okay if I take over her sessions until she is feeling better. Bill agrees; in this small town, word travels quickly when it comes to health. He knows that her back has been hurting but not about the tumors. Mom has insisted we not tell anyone, although I'm pretty sure Bill suspects it's more than just a sore back because I'm home.

After I work out, I drive to Riesbeck's, the downtown grocery store formerly called Pick-n-Save. I park in a space not far from the entrance and look over at the pickup truck next to me. There's a huge bloodhound with droopy eyes and ears in the passenger seat looking back at me through his raindrop-stained window. I love this dog and feel as if he somehow understands me. There's a sticker below the window in the shape of a paw that says "Who Rescued Who?" which makes me cry. I, too, want to be rescued. I imagine what my therapist, David, will say when I tell him about my desire to be rescued like a shelter dog, and I laugh because I already know the answer. I have to rescue myself. I look back at the dog and the sticker and realize it should say "Who Rescued *Whom*?" I turn my key in the ignition and move to a space farther out in the parking lot for a little more privacy from shoppers and their dogs.

I'm now facing west, looking right at the Pepsi distribution building. I used to go to that building back in high school to ask Dick Johnson, the CEO, to buy ads for the high school yearbook. I was the editor, of course, and Mr. Johnson would make me come into his office and tell him about my classes and where I wanted to go to college. Now it's twenty-seven years later, and I'm sitting here in my mom's green pickup truck waiting for 11:00 a.m. so I can call David. I didn't want to call from the farm because I worried about Mom hearing us talking about how hard it is waiting for the results of her blood work. Also, my phone doesn't always get reception there, down in the "holler" as the locals might say.

I've been talking to David for nearly five years, and while I know I've made some progress, I also know I'm going to need some help navigating whatever mode I'm in now. I've been thinking about how much change one woman can take and whether survival is the same as change.

My phone pings with a calendar notification. It's 11:00 a.m., and it's time to call David.

"This is David," he answers.

"Hi, David. It's Sarah," I say, which is how we start every session by phone since I left New York. I wonder if we'll ever drop this formality, but I've gotten used to it. When I would meet him in person, he would stand to greet me each time I walked through the door, and this verbal exchange has taken the place of our previous in-person ritual.

Our sessions often start with some banter until I'm ready to get into the harder stuff. David usually waits for me to dive in, or if I'm quiet, he simply asks me what's on my mind.

Today, I start before he has to ask.

"David, I really don't know what I'm supposed to be doing. I'm glad I'm here with Mom, but seriously, for fuck's sake. I don't have a job. I don't even have an apartment anymore. I don't know if I can handle Mom dying, and she's really sick. How am I supposed to figure all of this out and be strong for her? I feel like I'm going to let her down."

I'm not crying yet, and I haven't even told him about that damn rescue dog.

"Let's go slowly," he says. "There's a lot happening right now. See if you can tell me what part upsets you most."

David is calm, each word intentional, and his voice soothes me the same way a big exhale helps you get ready for your next breath. And so our parking-lot therapy begins.

HOW THERAPY STARTED

I remember the night I emailed David about working together. It was 2012 and I was sitting in my office in New York. I was the chief marketing officer at Girl Scouts of the USA, and I tried to stay in the office until my entire team had gone home at the end of the day. Terrible pop music—my favorite—was playing through my computer speakers, and I'd found sixteen other things to do while the draft sat open, staring at me as I contemplated hitting send. I wasn't afraid of therapy per se. I didn't think less of people who saw therapists; I just didn't fall for that cliché of bored women with too much time and money who created problems that didn't actually exist to give them something to do for an hour every week. I knew therapy helped so many people, but I was frightened about what I might find out.

More than anything, I was terrified that I would learn that there was no way to fix me, that the way I felt was just how I was going to feel for the rest of my life.

I'd turned forty that summer. I celebrated on Nantucket with my college pals. We rented a big, beautiful home a few minutes from Main Street for a week. I made paella for all of us on the first night. I had gotten some funny looks on the flight from LaGuardia, me with my laptop and my enormous paella pan stuffed into an L.L.Bean tote. We sat outside on the patio smoking cigarettes and drinking too much wine, contemplating that we were, in fact, *forty*. We were astounded that we had lived this long and experienced so much even though we all admitted we still kind of felt like dumb twenty-year-olds stumbling out of the Pub, our favorite dive bar in college. Who decided we should be allowed to be grown-ups?

What my friends didn't know, and what I didn't tell them, was that after we all went to bed, I lay there with tears streaming down my face. I wasn't sobbing. There was no noise, just tears sliding out, rivulets of hot, salty liquid pooling into wet spots on the nice linen pillowcases with navy scalloped trim. I was crying because I knew that I couldn't take another forty years of feeling the way I felt. I couldn't make sense of it; I didn't know what caused the pain or where it came from. I disliked myself, and I was tired of the feelings that commanded so much of my energy, and the constant feedback loop of self-loathing that had been with me since childhood.

Therapy seemed like the only option. But what if it didn't help? I was so scared that after I sent the email, after I met David, after I talked to him for one, two, or twenty sessions, he might tell me that this was just life. And if that happened, well, then what? What the fuck was I going to do then?

I thought about how our first session might go, knowing he would ask me what I wanted to work on. I knew I had to tell him the truth. I had to tell him that I was hurting and had been hurting for as long as I could remember, and to the best of my ability, no matter how I looked at my life, with all of my good fortune of family and friends and with all of my accomplishments that the world kept applauding, I still felt like shit about myself. Over the previous decade, I'd read every book and psychology magazine I could get my hands on, trying to find a similar profile to mine—*The Noonday Demon, Prozac Nation, Girl, Interrupted*—but I couldn't find an experience that matched. I didn't think I was suffering from depression, and I didn't think I needed to be medicated. I just wanted to feel better and stop the running tape on a loop telling me that I was a failure.

The problem I wanted to fix was *me*.

I finally sent the email.

David agreed to meet the next week.

***

My office was just ten blocks away from David's. Navigating New York City during rush hour in winter is like a sport, bumping against oversize down jackets and avoiding the thick, gray sludge of yesterday's snow. People's breath and taxi exhaust wrapped into one another over the jarring honks when somebody "blocked the box," the term New Yorkers use to mean pulling too far into an intersection. Determined commuters sprinted across anyway, ignoring the traffic and crosswalk signals as they headed home, and I headed to my first therapy session.

The Marble Collegiate Church was on the corner of his block, where I turned right on Twenty-Ninth Street. The fence around the church was covered with bright satin ribbons—gold and orange and yellow—commemorating soldiers who were killed in battle. They were long and beautiful and brilliant, creating a wall that shimmered in the winter wind, and they made me feel like I was in some sort of Sarah-Goes-to-Therapy parade.

My friend Elaine, also a therapist, recommended David. She explained that he was a Jungian therapist. I hadn't done any research on types of therapy, but I knew if I didn't want to be medicated, it likely would involve a lot of talking about things that weren't easy to talk about in the first place. Elaine described the focus on the conscious and unconscious parts of the mind, the striving to help patients feel balanced and whole. I didn't comprehend most of what she said, but I trusted her, wanted help, and found myself headed up to the fourth floor in a rickety elevator with the old-school black buttons you had to push really hard for the metal box to start moving.

I wondered if I would see another patient coming out of his office and worried that I would start sweating profusely after being bundled up from my walk. He opened the door and held out his hand. His handshake felt as if it was more than just a greeting, and more like an agreement that this would be okay. He had gray hair and a medium build and was older than me but not old-man old, and he was wearing a blue suit that was maybe a size too big. He had sweet eyes and the face of somebody I might be able to trust.

The room was small, with a dark blue sofa against the wall to the right, a small coffee table in front of it, and two windows on the wall across from the door. I sat down, and he pulled a chair over from the desk that was against the other wall and sat facing me with his legs crossed.

"I'm glad you're here, Sarah," he said.

"Thank you," I said, fidgeting a bit. "I'm really nervous, but I'm glad too."

"What are you nervous about?"

"I don't know, just all of it. But I really don't want to feel this way anymore."

"I think it's good that you reached out to me, and it's possible that this could help, but we'll have to see. Does that sound reasonable to you?"

"Well, yes, I mean, I'm here, right?" My sarcasm came out when I needed relief from the stress of admitting that I needed help.

"Yes, you are here. And that's something you should be pretty proud of in and of itself, that you're here at all."

That's when the tears started. Hearing him suggest that I should be proud of myself while knowing I could never feel truly proud of myself—or even good about myself—in any real way marked the exact coordinates on a map of my issues. I knew I had done things to be proud of, things in school, at work, and in life that other people responded to and praised me for, but it never added up. What had brought me to David was the frustration of feeling like shit even though my life was so good. And that made me feel worse about myself, and that made me cry even more.

There was a box of Kleenex on the table, and I thought maybe I should buy him a new box because I was using too many on day one. I wasn't watching the time, but it felt like the first full hour was me just sitting there crying, and David sitting there watching me cry.

"I can see this is really painful for you, so take the time you need," he said gently.

"Okay," I said, sniffling. "I'm sorry for all of the crying."

"Crying happens here sometimes," he replied. A little smile came to his lips and a slight tilt to his head, and I saw a twinkle in those kind eyes behind his glasses. He was making me feel comfortable, relieving the tension, making space for me to breathe.

"I'll bet it happens," I said. "But it's not a very good use of money to sit here and cry the whole time, is it?"

David smiled. I wanted him to like me. I wanted to make him laugh.

I knew there would be a lot of talking, if only I could stop crying. I couldn't place the cause of the tears—I didn't know whether I was crying because I was relieved to have a space to let the pain out or because I was so afraid this wouldn't help. During that first session, I noticed he didn't take notes, and I asked him about his process. I liked a good goal, so I really wanted to know how we would be able to tell if I was making progress.

He told me that the sessions would be spent discussing whatever was on my mind, that sometimes it might be something that had happened that week, or even that day, and that certain themes might come to light.

"I'm not here to give you answers," he said. "My expertise is to help guide you through understanding why you might be feeling a certain way, try to recognize patterns, and come up with tools to help you manage some of those feelings."

I liked his intelligence but wondered how he could remember anything if he didn't take notes. He could have fourteen other forty-year-old patients who cried while sitting on his sofa; how on earth would he keep us all straight? I told him I had one request that I hoped would be okay with him. If not, I wasn't sure this was going to work. I was crying again, the tears sliding down my jawline into the neck of my black cashmere sweater. More Kleenex.

"What is the request?"

"I'm not going to blame my parents for all of this."

"Okay, tell me more about what you mean."

"I have been so lucky in my life," I said, taking a breath. "My parents are smart and kind and generally pretty wonderful people. I'm not going to spend my time figuring out what they did or didn't do to make me this way. Too many people blame their parents for everything, and I'm just not going to do it. I am the way I am because of me, and I need to figure out how to fix all of this."

David nodded. He understood what I was saying.

"Let's see how the next few sessions go, and then we'll take it from there. How does that sound to you?"

I nodded back at him, collected my things, and left his office.

As I walked west on Twenty-Ninth Street after my session, the city humming around me and the cold night air on my still-hot face, I felt the tiniest stab of something strange, but good.

ABOUT THERAPY

You know I made it from the farm and then back again. There were big jobs and big cities and life stuff that happened in between. And now you also know that somewhere along the way I filled myself up with a whole shit ton of self-loathing. I'm going to show you some of that hard stuff—the anorexia stuff, the striving-for-gold-stars stuff—and my inability to find an ounce of self-worth even though I kept giving the world what I thought it wanted.

Some of these details matter because I became so good at hiding the pain from other people—and in some way, even from myself. I hid my suffering so well that my life looked fairly sparkly from the outside. But that's the thing about pain: it becomes part of who you are, not only in you but on you, a layer of skin you so badly want to shed but at the same time makes you who you are. I'm writing all of this down to try to make sense of things, and I trust my memory at least most of the time.

I'm not certain of the order of things, but I know one thing for sure: my current life wouldn't be possible without the work of therapy, which is why you're going to read about that part. Nobody wants to hear about my fucking therapy or your fucking therapy—the only thing worse is people talking about their dreams—but therapy changed the direction of my life. No, that's too passive. Therapy changed my life. Period.

You also need to know that there are going to be some poems along the way, starting now.

HOW WE BRUISE

First, there is contact,
the impact.
There is the thing hitting the thing
that must be our body
but probably is our heart.
This is how we bruise.
There is pain,
a stab and the wince and
awareness.
This thing has happened.
I am hurt.
Our bodies tell us that we hurt
before we wonder
how healing happens.
The pain is the warning,
a billboard that shouts pay attention
to this spot, look, do you see?
This thing has happened.
The bruise starts to shape.
A stain on the body.
A report written in past tense.
How big and what color?

The bruise wants to know how quickly you will
    forget
this thing has happened.
We feel the bruise to remind ourselves.
The same fingertips
create comfort
or pain.
The pressure of human touch.
Reds turn to yellow,
then brown like a leaf ready to fall.
We believe we are safe.
But life is all collision
until we learn how we bruise.

THE GRADES THING

Dad and Jane were at the kitchen table.

The kitchen table was also the dining table and homework table. It was an old butcher's table that still had the tally marks from how many steers or hogs had been butchered on it before it retired and ended up at Salt Creek Farm. It was a soft wood, and if you pressed too hard with your pencil, brown stains would show up on the back of the blue-lined school paper, an imprint of your time and effort.

I honestly don't know how old I was or what year it was. Jane is four years older than me, and she and Dad were working on math homework. I know there were multiplication tables, so Jane must have been nine or ten, in fourth grade perhaps, which means I was five or six. I was sitting in the living room where the TV was, likely looking at a picture book. It was a straight shot down the hall, and I could see Jane's back and Dad's profile. I don't know where Mom and Joe were; I just know the house was quiet aside from Jane and Dad's exchanges from the kitchen that seemed to go on forever.

"Jane, you know how to do this."

"I don't, Dad. I don't."

"Okay, let's start over. Look at the numbers where we started."

"I *am*."

"You're not. You're not paying attention to what I'm saying."

I could hear Dad's frustration, hear him saying things more slowly, not yet getting louder, just madder, more forceful in tone. Jane was also upset.

"I am paying attention. I just don't know the answer. It's too hard."

"It's not too hard. You're not trying. Jane, you have to try!"

I could hear her start to cry, and I could feel my own face getting hot.

"Okay, Janie, let's start over. Let's just start with two times two. Don't worry about the other part of the problem. It's easy. What is two times two?"

"I don't know."

Jane was trying to control her crying. Her back was to me down the hallway, but I could see her thin shoulders moving up and down, hunching up with each breath in and down again as she tried to get the breath out. Their voices got louder.

"YOU DO KNOW. JUST ANSWER THE QUESTION. WHAT IS TWO TIMES TWO? JESUS CHRIST, JANE."

"I DON'T KNOW, I DON'T KNOW!" she yelled back, and then in a quieter voice I heard her say, "Please stop yelling at me."

"I'm sorry, honey. I'm sorry for yelling, but I know you know how to do this."

By this time I was crying too, wanting it to be over. I pulled my knees into my chest and rocked. "Just say four," I whispered to myself. "Just say four. Just tell him what he wants to hear. Jane, say four. Please say four. Say four."

I wanted Jane to be out of pain. And I wanted Dad not to be so upset. I knew that if she told him the answer he wanted, things would get better.

Dad relented. I saw him touch the top of her head, stroking her pretty reddish-brown hair and telling her it was going to be okay. Then they stopped, or at least took a break.

I don't know what happened next—if Mom took over and tried again later that night or the next morning over breakfast. Jane liked runny eggs and cantaloupe, so maybe Mom sat with her quietly and helped her finish the math problems before she got on the school bus.

What I do know is that right then, I figured out how simple it would be to make my parents happy.

A FEW WORDS ON DAD

After a scene like that one, you might wonder why there isn't more of Dad in this book. If so, you're not alone, because he'd be pissed he isn't more of a star here. He deserves his own book, but this one isn't about him. Here's the deal: our relationship was uncomplicated and easy and certainly simpler than the one I had with Mom.

I didn't have to untangle myself from Dad, so he doesn't get a lot of memoir real estate. But still, I want you to know some things about him, because he was one of the coolest people I've ever known.

TEN TRUE THINGS ABOUT DAD

1. He had a best friend from childhood who was blind, and Dad let him drive his car while providing coaching from the passenger seat. When the friend spoke at Dad's funeral, he told us Dad could have been a better copilot.
2. He wrote a poem in college called "All Women Are Whores," which I realized later was a feminist commentary on how few choices women in his generation had.
3. He loved kids. Adored kids. Taught them to eat French fries with mustard and shout "oui oui" as loud as they could to celebrate each bite.
4. He thought farming was the purest form of work.
5. He was smart as shit but not a braggart or remotely condescending unless he thought somebody was an asshole—and then whammo, get ready for a Joe Gormley zinger.
6. He didn't talk about heroes, but Jack Nicholson and Willie Nelson were his kind of men.
7. Thought the perfect meal would be two martinis and a hot fudge sundae.
8. Had a kidney transplant at age forty. Never once complained, but all of the meds were hard on his body. His kidney kept functioning until he died an awful,

unconscionable death thirty-five years later when he was starved to death while hopped up on morphine in a hospice facility. I have a huge right-to-die rant, but this is not that book, either. Still. We should be able to do fucking better.

9. He called Mom "honey," always asked her for a kiss when he walked in the door, and once told me that even though she wasn't the easy choice, marrying her was the best decision he ever made.

10. He made lists on yellow legal pads we would find all over the house.

On his first official day in the office after being sworn in as Judge Gormley, Dad left this note on the kitchen table for Mom—on a yellow legal pad.

As further proof of my theory that no matter what happened yesterday, tomorrow will occur . . . Here it is, 7:45 on what is arguably the most important day of my career, and you and Calvin are still in bed.

Calvin was a ninety-five-pound Doberman.

GATEWAYS TO SUCCESS

From the kitchen scene on, the thing that became most important to me, from as early as elementary school, was the report card—proof of how I compared to others. "Satisfactory" was what I wanted to avoid. I was always looking for an S+ or even an S++, usually with handwritten commentary about how well I had done. I knew when the report cards would show up in the mail and could feel the anticipation of seeing how I had performed. I needed to make sure I was better than the rest—ideally, the best student in the class. Although my parents didn't reward us or even express overt praise when the report cards came, I knew the grades were a measure of me, and if something could be measured, I knew what success looked like.

And then the standardized tests came. Schools didn't share those scores as easily. In fact, my parents didn't seem willing to talk about them when my siblings and I had to take them. In hindsight, I am sure they were trying to protect Jane, who continued to struggle in school, while my brother and I quickly became part of the "gifted" groups.

But I knew where they kept those forms. The official-looking envelopes with the computer-generated reports with charts and black dots with numbers that correlated to aptitude and intelligence quotient. They were like secret CIA documents that held the secrets of our identities, and I was obsessed with them.

Those papers lived in the top drawer of a large antique dresser in Mom and Dad's bedroom.

Even as the tallest girl in fourth grade, I couldn't touch the top two drawers. There was a blue floral wingback chair and a small drop-leaf table to the right, and I knew how to climb up, perched with one foot on the back of the chair, one foot on the arm, so I could get to the top, reach my hand in, and fish around until I felt the paperwork. Then I could lift it out with one hand while the other hand pressed into the front of the dresser so I could balance and inch down without toppling out of the chair. I would time the dresser climbs so I could take the forms upstairs to study the dots and numbers for ten to fifteen minutes and then replace them before Mom came back into the house.

The dots and charts reassured me. Permanently recorded on paper, official numbers that told me I was exceptional, which I so badly wanted to be true.

THE WEIGHT THING

The weight thing started years later with a number on a Post-it note at summer camp. Brown Ledge Camp (BLC) was and still is an unusual, independence-first girls' camp in Vermont, which became known as "snob camp" in my family given my stories about some of the other campers' affluent backgrounds. These girls were decidedly *not* farm girls. I went to BLC for four summers and was a junior counselor when I stuck the first yellow square on the graffitied cabin wall, just above my cot and next to pictures of my family and our pets, and a photo of Shawn Harper (my quarterback crush from high school who had never spoken to me). I wrote down my first number that night after dinner, before my friend Betsy and I went for our usual evening walk.

That's how it started. I had just turned sixteen, and I decided to lose weight.

I wasn't overweight—not even close. I was five feet eight inches with a body type that magazines called "athletic," and I was lean and muscular. My riding instructors often commented about my leg strength and how well I could hold a two-point position, which is when you hover over the saddle. But my hip bones didn't jut out of my shorts, my thighs often touched, and when I sat down I could feel the skin of my tummy fold over my jeans a little bit.

The first number on a Post-it was 142.

I wasn't one of the skinny girls.

I started observing what and how some of the older counselors ate, and copied them. Less granola at breakfast. Skim milk. Salad for lunch. Always salad for lunch. No dessert—unless it was fruit or a small serving of vanilla yogurt. BLC was the kind of camp where an actual baker made fresh bread every day—gorgeous light-brown-crusted loaves lined up on the counter waiting to be served and enjoyed by activity-exhausted campers. I stopped spreading already-melting butter on the warm bread because Annie, who was a riding counselor, never actually ate the bread. She would pick pieces off of the edges and pop them into her mouth, then cover her mouth with her hand as she chewed the tiny brown specks. Annie was thin.

The scale outside the nurse's station was the kind they had at doctors' offices, with the little weight you slide over to the right. Push it too far and down it went with a clank, but when you hit the right weight the bar balanced just so, hovering in place, suspended in quiet certainty. I loved the exactness of that scale—it was not one of those small square ones you step on and kind of squint at to guess where the red arrow hits.

This scale told you the truth.

Nobody noticed, and I don't recall talking about the diet or the numbers. But I loved the anticipation of stepping onto that scale and the payoff of seeing smaller numbers that I would then write on the Post-it, my makeshift ledger. There were days that the number stayed flat, but the trajectory was downward overall, and that sense of accomplishment was glorious.

Those last few weeks at camp were the start of something I could do to better fit my idea of success. My decision to lose weight was entirely pragmatic: this is what the world wants and what gets rewarded; therefore, I will be skinny.

I knew I could achieve more by being less.

BEING GOOD AT SOMETHING

There was no better feeling than lying flat in the bathtub to see how little water it took to cover my hip bones. Anorexia is rewarding that way, with visual markers of success. Mom always preferred baths to showers, so she hadn't put a shower upstairs when they put an addition on the house. So even though most mornings I would traipse downstairs to shower in Dad's bathroom (where the second weigh-in of the day took place), some evenings I would take a bath just for the counting. I counted how many minutes it took for the hot water from the faucet to fully cover my abdomen and then crest over the peaks of my hip bones. That last part, coming over my hip bones, added at least forty-five seconds to the total time.

I was a really good anorexic. That's what people don't seem to understand—that it feels so good to be so good at something. The starving nourished me and filled me up; the rituals of those days felt better than any bite of a chocolate cupcake, and I found satisfaction in checking the mirrors to make sure I hadn't gotten any bigger.

There was a mirror on the door in my bedroom. The first step on the scale was always after I peed, because every ounce of everything counts when it comes to the scale. Then into the walk-in closet with white carpet and mirrors covering the walls and ceilings I went. The irony was that Mom had surprised me when I got home from camp by redoing what had been my childhood playroom, because I loved modern design and architecture. She wanted me to have something of my own, something that felt like my style rather than the style of the 1800s farmhouse, but she had no idea that those mirrors would become part of such a destructive routine.

I typically did thirty to fifty pliés after I took off my pajamas to make sure I could see my legs, butt, and stomach, ensuring they were firm and thin, that they hadn't betrayed me overnight by getting softer or bigger. Then downstairs to shower, and another scale—this one was digital—because I liked to have a number to compare against the one upstairs to be sure.

Just to be sure.

And of course, there was the eating part. I used eating to prove to myself and others that I was fine. In the morning before school, it was a half cup of Special K, with just enough skim milk to wet the cereal: 125 calories to start the day and then off to school. Lunch in the cafeteria consisted of four ounces of orange juice (50 calories), two saltines (17 calories each), and a salad with no dressing, no cheese, and only the white part of two hard-boiled eggs (40 calories). More counting, always keeping it under 400 until approaching the challenge of dinner.

My friends typically were on some type of diet too, or at least they claimed to be, and while people sometimes commented on how skinny I was, nobody seemed worried. Mainly because I wasn't somebody you worried about. That was all part of the storyline: Sarah Gormley got all As; Sarah Gormley was the yearbook editor; Sarah Gormley would sure as shit be valedictorian; and oh yes, Sarah Gormley is skinny. That too.

After lunch, during study hall, I'd go down to the girls' locker room to weigh myself again on the doctor-style scale, and before I left I would always, always climb up on the bench near the sinks to check my hips bones in the mirror. I would unzip and pull down my jeans so I could see the bones pressing out against my underwear. I needed to see them to make sure I was still skinny.

Just to be sure.

The rituals and the counting calmed me. I felt responsible, powerful, and in control. There's a sublime intimacy to anorexia—you're relying on yourself and your body not to give in, to be strong. Something I've never admitted to anyone else is that after so many hours of no calories, you're not actually hungry anymore. You kind of hit a plateau of emptiness, a numb state that makes it easier not to eat. But I'd sometimes make a snack—a bite, really—that was just enough to remind my stomach of its job, to feel the digestive system kick in, to feel the stabs of hunger that came from even a few pretzel sticks in what was an empty, hollow vessel.

I wanted to feel the pain of hunger so I could feel the pleasure of denying it.

I wanted to succeed.

WHEN A SETBACK IS A WARNING

When senior year started, I weighed 106 pounds. I had lost almost a third of my body weight in eighteen months, and clothes draped over me, hanging on to my collarbones and hip bones. My body was like one of those jointed wooden models used by students learning to draw, the angular forms and shapes creating the outline of a human being.

The pecan rolls were in the cabinet where Mom kept the plates. They were breakfast treats for people who ate breakfast treats. Not me. I didn't eat anything, certainly not little round spirals of carbohydrates and brown sugar, not at ninety calories and six fat grams apiece.

It was a Thursday night, and I had a paper for Dr. Lepp due the next day. I'd received nothing lower than an A– from Dr. Lepp, the quirky English teacher at podunk Philo High School, where we considered ourselves lucky to have a teacher with a PhD. For whatever reason, the draft of the paper on Faulkner wasn't where it needed to be for me to finish it for class the next morning, and my heart was racing. The paper would account for 15 percent of my final grade and had to be an A.

I paced between the front room of the farmhouse, where the nightly news was on, and the kitchen, where the pots hung from a metal rack on the wooden boards of the ceiling. I walked back and forth, taking small sips of water every other trip, contemplating if I should eat something.

Thursdays were generally okay days if I made it that far in the week without a slipup on calories. My counting included the days of the week, and one bad move—part of a sleeve of saltines, the indulgence of Italian dressing on a salad on Monday—could throw a wrench in the entire week. This one had been fine so far, and I'd skipped the salad and saltines at lunch to make up for the calories spent on the extra half cup of Special K I'd allowed myself at breakfast. I had a baked potato with Molly McButter—some powdery substance, not butter at all—for dinner so I was at no more than six hundred calories so far, and I was determined to make it to bed without giving in.

But I couldn't write, couldn't sit down and get the words on the page, so my mind raced between scenarios where I got an incomplete and a lower grade because I now didn't have time to make it A quality. If I didn't get the A, would it throw off the grade for the term, possibly pushing into the final grade for the semester, even into the 4.0 grade point average I'd maintained for four years?

I couldn't calm myself down. It was just me and Ben, the first of the two enormous and sweet Dobermans we had, asleep in his bed in the corner (who had probably been wondering why I was pacing) until my parents got home from dinner.

I thought about a bite of something to calm me. Just one.

But I kept taking more bites on this particular night until I ate three entire ninety-calorie pecan rolls and felt my world start to fall apart. It wasn't a panicked, binge-like consumption. It was slow and methodical. And I wouldn't dare vomit, as bulimia was for people who couldn't control themselves. The hierarchy of eating disorders is unspoken but fascinating, and it pains me now to think how little sympathy I had for other girls who were suffering. I thought bulimia was for the weak—people who had to binge for comfort and then expel what became their own disgust. Anorexics were all about control, not giving in, fighting our disdain by trying to dominate it with denial. Neither method rids you of your self-hatred, but there would be no puking for me.

I knew I would have to wait it out and start the next day at zero calories, but I couldn't get my heart to stop racing and my hands to stop shaking before I saw the headlights coming up the driveway. I knew my parents would know something was wrong, and I was so ashamed by the thought of them seeing me this way because I thought they wanted me to be perfect, and perfection didn't include this kind of meltdown.

Mom walked in the door first.

"Hi, honey . . . how was your night? Did you finish the paper?"

"No, I couldn't do it . . . I couldn't write it this time," I said, my voice cracking.

Dad walked in behind Mom, confused by the tears that had started flowing, streaking down the sides of my hot face. I was no longer able to talk, trying to gulp in breaths, wishing they didn't have to see me falling apart.

"Let's go out here and sit down for a little bit, and you can try to tell us what's going on," said Mom.

I followed Mom into the front room. She pulled me into her lap, the way I used to sit with her when I was a little girl when we watched *Another World* together after I got home from kindergarten. She stroked my back until I was breathing somewhat normally again, the sobs tapering off. It felt like hours—at least long enough for one TV show to end and something else to begin, maybe the news again. I could feel the comfort of her hands, her skin, and her breath on the back of my neck and wanted to be small again, to start over somehow.

I told them I didn't know what had happened, that I just couldn't write the paper. I didn't tell them about the pecan rolls because I felt such shame, not only for eating them but also for being so weak.

Looking back, I think this was the first of a series of breakdowns in my life. "Breakdown" sounds much bigger than what I permitted myself to believe had happened at the time, because I could barely admit to myself that something was wrong. Is a breakdown defined by how you feel or how you are treated? Do you need a diagnosis to make it real?

There were no hospital stays or doctors in white coats, but these were specific breaking points in time when the years and months and days and minutes of self-loathing and striving to please and achieve and succeed needed an outlet. It felt like lifting the lid off of something boiling to release some of the steam before closing the lid again, when you know the boiling will continue but you're somehow avoiding—or postponing—the really big explosion.

And even in this suffering that I couldn't yet name, there was something that upset me even more.

What I feared most was the possibility that by allowing my parents to see me hurt, I would in turn cause them pain, and that was unbearable to me. What I didn't know yet was that from a young age, I was so focused on pleasing them that my real identity didn't have a chance to fully form. My commitment to becoming the right version of me was so strong that I actually succeeded.

SKINNY WAS A WAY OF LIFE

I grew up through Mom's diets. When she was on Atkins, we went to the chain steak house Ponderosa so she could get a rib eye for lunch. The lady behind the register always gave me a Tootsie Pop when we left, and I liked the ones in the blue wrapper best.

Here's the thing: I always thought Mom was beautiful and would have thought so no matter what, but she was always thin. I never saw her remotely heavy or overweight. She was different from other moms for sure, because she didn't wear makeup and didn't wear jewelry, as if she was forcing you to see her as she really was. And we loved her for it. Everyone loved Susan Gormley.

Her style was her attitude—not giving a fuck about things that didn't matter. But even with her abundance of Susan-Gormley-ness, she always wanted to lose weight. What I learned and what society reinforced was that Mom wasn't a beautiful woman who happened to be thin; she was a beautiful woman *because* she was thin.

Mom coached us to suck in our stomachs as little girls, explaining that if we started young we could have flat stomachs for the rest of our lives. I don't know if she said it many times or only once on the way home from the pool where we saw my friend Bethany with her seven-year-old tummy poking out after too many frozen Snickers from the refreshment stand.

"Girls, I'm going to tell you something, and you're going to think I'm crazy," she started.

We just looked at her, not knowing what she was trying to say.

"You know how I look in my bathing suit?"

We did. It was a bright blue one-piece, conservative by today's standards, but with a deep scoop at the neckline and tight all over, hugging her tiny waist.

"Well, I look good because I watch my weight, but I also suck in my stomach all of the time," she said. "That's the secret. You just have to keep your belly tight, and if you start doing it now, you'll always have a flat stomach. Clothes will look better on you, and you'll feel better about yourself. You probably think I'm nuts, but you'll remember me telling you this one day, and you'll be happy I told you."

At the time, I was probably wishing I had another frozen Snickers for the ride home, but her advice did stick with me, and I started sucking in my stomach even as a little girl.

Weight mattered, and if somebody was fat, it was almost as bad as if they were lazy, in debt, or didn't go to college. Especially for women. I don't recall Dad ever commenting on his big-bellied, borderline-obese golf buddies, but I knew which of their wives were too heavy. We didn't need magazines to tell us the world liked women who were thin better because we heard it over and over at the kitchen table on Clay Pike. It was pragmatic, really, or it seemed that way in our family. Society seemed to prefer women who were thin, so we should be thin.

This is why things got difficult for Jane, who struggled with her weight in high school. Or at least we *assumed* she struggled because she wasn't naturally thin, and in our house, of course you wanted to be thin. When I found Dexatrim pills in her dresser her senior year, I wondered if Mom knew about them, but I also thought Mom likely was happier if Jane was thin, no matter how she got that way. We grew up in the same house, but Jane and I were different. I think she used food for comfort, what doctors might call emotional eating, and I took the opposite approach. I found comfort in hunger and the feeling of emptiness.

LOOKING FOR CAUSES

I'm choosing which scenes to share and putting them in a particular order, because it turns out there's no other way to write a book. You choose what words to put down on the page. You hope they make sense. You commit the words to a certain order to convey what happened, but I'm afraid the order will make you think the scenes are causes.

Maybe I'm trying to protect my dead parents because I'm no good at blaming anybody but myself for anything. They wanted us to get good grades, and my mom wanted me to be skinny, so I got good grades and stayed skinny.

Smart, skinny, successful. That was the blueprint.

But wasn't that the blueprint society handed all of us, especially girls? Was Mom any different than any other Tab-drinking, Atkins-dieting mom who wanted her kids to succeed?

What I am trying to figure out is why I reacted to my set of circumstances the way I did. How did I come through the things that happened in a certain way and begin to reorder them? Sometimes what you believe are causes are really just symptoms waiting for a cause to emerge.

THE COONER

Even after the doctor's appointment and seeing how poorly she felt, I refused to accept that this Thanksgiving might be our last one with Mom.

Thanksgiving was the holiday made to be celebrated at the farm.

Of course, there was the setting: the black farmhouse up on the hill with the pond down below. The hills and the tree lines curved to the east and west, framing the property more than the fence line did. The crisp oranges and reds of fall leaves gave way to frost, and the breath from the cattle rose like steam near the round bales Joe put out for them in the morning.

The Cooner is a hunt for raccoons. A group of men, all wearing Carhartts and headlamps, march into the dark woods on foot or on their buggies—those sport utility vehicles sometimes called side-by-sides, which basically can take you anywhere a normal truck can't go—with barking hound dogs to hunt for raccoons. The dogs tree the raccoon, and then something happens with a spotlight. Maybe it scares the raccoon and it freezes? From what I've been told, there's only one rifle and whoever is selected to be the marksman attempts to shoot the raccoon out of the tree.

The hunting part is only the *putative* purpose for the Cooner.

The real reason for the Cooner, which started nearly thirty years ago, is that sometimes, some men want to get away from the stress of a family holiday. There's no formal documentation on this rationale, but it's a pretty good guess. After the Macy's parade, rounds of too much food, and football watching wherein the wrong team always wins, these men head into the woods. They head into the woods where the sounds are simple, primal even: breath in cold air, footsteps, dogs barking, the clear and air-parting sound of a gunshot. These sounds are their poetry one night of the year, and the night is almost theirs alone, but it also belongs to Susan Gormley.

Mom *loved* the Cooner. After her nap, we would watch the local news, then maybe have a turkey sandwich and a glass of Chardonnay while we waited for the men to show up for a break in the action. This is how it happened every year. She would see the headlamps down in the field and yell to Dad and me, "Here they come . . . Here come the Cooners . . . Get the whiskey!" with a level of excitement more commonly associated with little kids at Christmas.

The core group was my brother, our neighbors Bill and Brad McLoughlin, their cousin Camillus, and other guys from the "neighborhood" that spanned ten miles. As the years passed, invitations were extended to neighbors and college buddies, anyone who was visiting that year, and then the men who returned to Ohio specifically to participate, including a young Parisian who became "Frenchie," but of course. There are definitely knit hats and probably some T-shirts commemorating the Cooner. When we look back at photos, we try to recall what year it was based on who was in attendance and argue about who did what, in what order.

Mom and Dad held court, but especially Mom. She would happily explain the reason she loved the night so much was "all of these gorgeous boys in my kitchen, one cuter than the next." She called them boys even though most of them were married with children of their own. She quizzed each one to find out who he was (in the case of newbies) and whether life was going well. She would jokingly tell at least one or two of them they were an asshole for some type of infraction they confessed to her during this ceremony.

***

One of my favorite Cooner memories involved Camillus Musselman, Dad's brand-new buggy, and a muddy excursion down by the cave.

I had just started working for Martha Stewart in 2010 and became an easy target around the kitchen table that night. I was always there, year after year, and these guys enjoyed hearing my stories from New York even if they didn't quite understand why anyone would ever *choose* to live in such a place, especially when you could be right here in this idyllic setting.

Dad hadn't been feeling well and was resting in the bedroom. He never wanted to burden us or lessen anyone's fun because of his ongoing health challenges, and I'm sure he loved hearing the sounds of our laughter snaking through the farmhouse.

The week before, my brother picked up a brand-new buggy that Dad had bought for the farm, but really bought for *himself*. He was a man who liked toys, and when the Dodge minivan replaced the Cadillacs and the midlife-crisis, cringe-inducing red Corvette, he didn't have much room for more purchases. Hence, the buggy out in the barn, which Joe insisted wasn't to be driven until Dad started feeling better and had a chance to take it out on the farm himself.

"I thought about taking it out tonight for the Cooner but, hey, the thing is his, so he should be the first one to drive it," said Joe. "Those are the rules."

I'd known Camillus long enough and heard enough stories about him to know that he would be able to make a case for taking a test drive. A natural charmer with a big smile and sparkly eyes, he had probably convinced lots of people to do all sorts of things over the course of his life.

"Come on, man," he said to my brother. "Your dad didn't buy that thing so it would sit out there in the barn. Those things need to be driven. I think he would want one of us to take it out tonight and give it a test run."

The other guys laughed and looked at Mom, who gestured that she was staying out of this.

"No way," said Joe. "It's been raining for three days, and you know what will happen if somebody takes it out—it will end up stuck or wrecked and he'll be pissed. And we all know better than to piss off The Judge."

It felt like a conclusion for a few beats, but then Camillus looked right at me.

"The Judge wouldn't care if Sarah takes it out . . . She never does anything wrong."

I looked at him and then looked at Joe, and in a move that surprised everyone in the room, I told Camillus that I would take the buggy out, but only if he came with me.

"Okay, big talker, let's go," I said. "I just need to borrow some Carhartts."

Camillus jumped up to go get the buggy, while I assessed who was the smallest guy there and convinced him to take off his Carhartts so I could avoid getting covered in mud. It was pissing down rain, and I walked out and climbed into the passenger seat to the cheers and taunts of the drunken peanut gallery inside.

Camillus drove that buggy as fast as he could down the driveway, across the bridge, and back toward the cave, and the mud and water were already up to the middle of the wheels. Even a novice like me knew the conditions were ripe for getting stuck, which would mean a shame-fueled walk back to the house and teasing for years to come. I was glad he was driving.

About a mile back into the woods, across streams and through dense trees, there's a cave with an overhang and waterfall you can drive up into. Camillus navigated up the slick stone and turned the engine off. The only sound was the rain hitting the plastic roof of the buggy and the water coming down through the cave.

Right then, in that moment, I felt a sense of calm.

Every drop of water suddenly reminded me of how alone we were, the two of us, away from the action back in the kitchen where they were passing around the Jack Daniel's, away from Dad not feeling well again, away from New York and another big job that would have me working around the clock. I was away. Away from *everything*. I felt like I was suspended in place and time, and now, all of these years later, I can still take myself back to that moment to calm myself.

Somehow this moment felt intimate, not because there was any intimacy between us—Camillus was now standing in the cave—but because we were in something together, absorbing the sound of the rain, the smell of the damp rocks, and the quiet of nature when you let yourself listen. I felt safe.

Camillus stood there looking at me as I sat in the driver's seat of the buggy looking back at him, aware. We didn't say anything, just sat in the stillness of this particular Thanksgiving night. Finally, I suggested we probably should head back to the house. He told me to drive, even as I protested that I'd never really driven one of these things.

His advice was clear: "Listen to me, Sarah. Do not take your foot off the gas. If the mud gets deep, you've just got to hammer it, and whatever you do, KEEP GOING!"

MOM'S LAST COONER

Seven years later, Thanksgiving felt different. And so did the Cooner.

Dad died the year before, and Mom was now battling cancer and didn't want to host the big family meal during the day, which we all understood. We went to my cousin Cara's to eat and then headed back home so Mom could rest up for what we all suspected might be her last Cooner.

We saw the men's headlamps down in the field just after dusk. I knew that they probably decided to come early in the hopes that Mom would feel well enough to sit at the kitchen table.

She mustered up enthusiasm even though I knew she felt like shit.

"Here they come, Sarah," she said. "Go get the whiskey."

She wanted to see the boys, and they wanted to see her. I didn't dare make eye contact with my brother, Bill, Brad, or Camillus because I knew I would start crying, which might tap into their own deep reservoirs of love for Mom.

I didn't want to ruin this moment for anyone.

I wanted Mom to have her favorite night of the year one more time.

TEN TRUE THINGS ABOUT MOM

1. Susan Cameron was the youngest of three. She had no middle name, as her parents thought she might want to keep Cameron if and when she got married.
2. When her parents attended her first dance recital—tap, I believe—the instructor suggested perhaps she should give up dancing and they should buy her a horse.
3. She ended up at Stephens College in Missouri because she wanted to get out of class when the representative had come to her high school. Mom thought a liberal arts degree sounded interesting but worried that she didn't know how to draw.
4. After a month of being terribly homesick, Grandpa Cameron decided to send something out to Stephens to cheer her up. He sent her horse.
5. She thought her career choices were secretary, teacher, or nurse. She chose to be a teacher and taught junior-high history before becoming a high school guidance counselor.
6. When they brought my sister home from the hospital, Mom saw a group of men hunting in the lower field and wanted more than anything to be out there rather than in the house with a newborn.

7. She once told me she didn't think she should have had children.

8. Grandma Cameron never told Mom she loved her. She did sign birthday and anniversary cards—the ones that always included a twenty-dollar bill—"Love, Mom," however.

9. Mom struggled with depression and started taking Prozac when diagnosed at age forty-five.

10. She believed a hot bath and a nap could cure just about anything.

FIRST CHEMO APPOINTMENT

When your mom has cancer in a small town like Zanesville, everyone knows.

I'm not sure if that's a good thing or a bad thing, but it made Mom crazy.

"I don't want anyone to know what's going on with me," Mom said. "Do you hear me?"

I was driving her to her first chemotherapy appointment, to the cancer center named after Nick and Nancy Sarap, who were family friends, and the volunteer who checked us in at reception recognized Mom from their high school class.

"I'm not sure we're going to be able to control who knows, considering your old pal Shirley just gave you your wristband," I said.

Mom didn't laugh. She raised the right side of her upper lip in one of the many facial expressions we used in what sometimes became a full dialogue without either of us saying a word.

- The raised nostril and lip combo meant "Yuck, I don't like what you just said."

- The raised nostril and lip combo with a nod meant "Yuck, I don't like what you just said, but I understand and accept what you just said."
- Two raised eyebrows and big eyes meant "I'm making fun of you by acting as if what you said is at all a surprise."
- A single-motion kiss face meant "I love you and want you to know."
- Multiple kisses in fast succession meant "I know you're mad but don't be mad."

We waited for Dr. Wegner in a small room. Two nurses came in, one to take Mom's temperature and blood pressure, the other to type on a laptop on the tall wheeled cart next to the small counter and sink in the corner.

We heard words like "metastasized" and "aggressive" and "lymph nodes," and I kept looking at Dr. Wegner rather than at Mom, afraid I might start crying. He told us the plan would be to start with two treatments: One was chemo she would get through an IV every other week. The other was a medication taken through two shots injected into her butt during the week without chemo, plus a regimen of pills to be taken at specific times. He told us we would try this for six weeks, and then he would do more blood work that would tell us whether her counts were improving. I liked how he said "we," which made me feel as though he was experiencing this with us. As he spoke, Mom was quiet but then blurted out a question.

"Can you tell me what you think my chances of survival are?"

He paused and then exhaled.

Mom and I knew this was bad news. But Dr. Wegner wasn't part of our club, so maybe he just wanted to be as clear as possible.

"Susan, I cannot tell you that right now," he responded. "I can tell you that we've put together the best possible treatment plan to fight the cancer, and we have to wait and see how your body reacts. The challenge will be managing the side effects and keeping some quality of life for you as we fight."

Mom and I raised our nostrils and lips as we nodded.

We understood.

***

When Mom had cancer the first time, she acted as if the disease did her a favor. I was living in Chicago, a few years out of college. I remember staying up all night to make her the perfect mixtape to help keep her mood lifted.

She was diagnosed with breast cancer postmenopause, opted for a double mastectomy, and agreed to be part of a trial for what we now believe was Tamoxifen. The surgery and recovery were rough, but Mom complained very little, if at all, while the tubes drained the orangey-red liquid and tissue from the incision sites and cavities where the tumors—and her flesh—once resided.

Mom always hated her "big boobs," as she called them. She claimed they made it difficult to look good in certain dresses, which really meant they made it difficult to look thin. I remember watching her cut the underwire out of the minimizer bras that she bought a size too small so she could "smash 'em down" and flatten them out. I've been thankful for my small boobs my entire life and honestly still tend to agree with her about the clothes thing.

She didn't have any reconstructive surgery and proudly wore swimsuits with little to no padding to celebrate her flat chest.

The first time she had cancer, Mom was the victor.

***

Mom insisted that I not sit with her for the ninety minutes of the first chemo session, telling me she wanted me to go have some lunch and come back to take her home because she knew her bed would be calling.

She had her phone, and I told her to text me if she changed her mind.

As I was walking out of the cancer center, I saw Dr. Hernandez, her primary care physician. He was Dad's doctor and known to be brusque and a little bit of an asshole, but he was also the best doctor in town. He adored Mom and Dad and told us that he kept a picture of Dad on his desk as a reminder of how tough he had been, how his stubborn will to live kept him alive for years.

He stopped when he saw me.

"Hi, Dr. Hernandez," I said. "Mom's starting chemo today. Her spirits seem to be okay, I think."

He put his hands on his hips and looked at the gray faux-marble floor, hesitating before making eye contact with me again.

"I just looked at her charts," he said. "It's bad. The numbers are terrible."

"But we have to try the treatment, right? We have to try something, don't we?"

"Yes, of course you should try, but I'm afraid she doesn't have anything left in her tank to fight. Her reserves are gone, Sarah. It's bad."

I don't know what I said or if I said anything at all.

I remember walking out of the hospital into the parking lot and gulping in the December air to remind myself I could still breathe. I promised myself that I wouldn't tell Mom or my siblings what Dr. Hernandez said because . . . well, Jesus fuck. Nobody wants to hear that shit. And yet, some part of me realized that Mom already knew she was dying and didn't need any doctor to explain that to her.

I now believe Mom only agreed to start any treatment at all because she wanted to make the rest of us feel better.

MEET CAMILLUS

One morning, weeks after I got back to Ohio, after the weird Thanksgiving night, after what may have been Mom's last Cooner, and after her first treatment, I passed Camillus Musselman on a blurry drive home from my friend Ali's house. I had slept over after I attempted to drink all of the red wine in Muskingum County the night before, and I felt like I might have succeeded.

Over July Fourth weekend earlier that year, before we even knew Mom was sick, Joe had jokingly suggested that I might "give Camillus a little bit of attention" the next time I was home. He was going through a divorce and could use the distraction, Joe said.

Because my mom might be dying, because I thought I might be having a nervous breakdown, because my head hurt from the bad decisions the night before, and because the thought of having somebody like Camillus to keep my mind off of all of *that* seemed like a great idea, I decided to listen to my brother.

I sent Camillus a text.

"Exactly how long am I going to have to be home before you ask me to go out?"

THE ORDER OF THINGS

The response came within minutes: "I'll pick you up in fifteen minutes."

His reply came so fast, actually, that I missed it at first. I was upstairs washing my face and brushing my teeth, trying to scrub away the red wine stains from the night before, so I didn't see his answer. I didn't even know Camillus had responded to my text until he was already standing in the front room waiting for me at 9:45 on that crisp December morning.

He told me he had some errands to run—had to buy a mattress, in fact—and that I should go with him. He said a quick hello to Mom, who was resting, and I told her I'd be back in a few hours.

Camillus and I hadn't been alone together since Thanksgiving in 2010, when we took Dad's new buggy out in the rain and the mud. As I climbed into his truck, I realized that although I didn't really know much about him at all, I liked his smile and figured that some sex with somebody as sparkly as Camillus might be good for my soul.

We'd been driving for a few minutes when I decided to just put it out there.

"Here's my deal, Camillus," I said, taking a breath. "I decided to take a year off of work no matter what happens because I thought I was about to have a nervous breakdown. So I'm a single forty-five-year-old living in her childhood bedroom. I have no job, no home, and no car. And I think Mom is probably going to die. My life is a fucking disaster. But I'm pretty smart, my friends think I'm funny, and I made a shit ton of money in San Francisco. So, yeah, that's me. Oh, and I can be a bit of a snob, you should know that."

He looked at me.

I didn't know his looks yet.

"Well, Sarah, here's my deal. I'm about to finalize a divorce, which has been pretty awful and the hardest thing I've ever gone through, but I have two amazing kids as a result, so my life's not a complete disaster. I do all right at work, and it might not be a shit ton, but I make enough money to pay the bills and to do the things I want to do. My friends at least act like they like me, and I like to have fun now and then."

We weren't yet five miles from the farm when I said what I said next. I didn't know what he would think and didn't care. I just knew I wanted to make this man laugh.

"I have a question for you."

"Okay, I happen to be taking questions at the moment, so go ahead, Sarah."

"Can you still fuck?"

Another look. A head tilt.

"Well." He paused. "Yeah, I think so. I can still fuck."

And then he smiled.

Right then, I didn't know that smile. His smile.

But what I did know as he drove us into town so he could buy a mattress was this:

1. My relationships never lasted more than three months.
2. Dad's death the year before was brutal, but Mom's death had the potential to unravel me for good.
3. While my work with David was helping me see myself in a new way, I still had no idea what to do next with my life.
4. The more successful I was in my career, the more miserable I became, and something had to change.
5. For the first time in my life, I didn't have the energy to be what I thought other people wanted me to be.

6. Camillus was seeing me at my worst, and somehow I didn't care.

***

The mattress was purchased off of Old Route 40 in some kind of warehouse/junk store I wasn't even sure we should be entering. I asked a few questions.

"Are we really going in there?"

"What makes you think they sell mattresses?"

"So this is where you should be buying a mattress?"

I feared he would already see the snob in me coming out, but I was also concerned there could very well be rabid dogs waiting to attack us at any minute. The place looked like a crime scene waiting to happen.

"Somebody told me this guy buys things that fall off Amazon trucks or whatever, so it's all in good shape aside from some ripped boxes, and it's all super cheap," he said.

Again, I wasn't sure that these things should be considered *positives* in the mattress-purchasing decision, but I decided to keep my mouth shut. Turned out that the guy did have some mattresses, one of which I flopped down on, turning to the right and then to the left the way you do in an actual mattress store, well aware that any woman rolling around on a mattress might be hinting at something sexual. But this situation was so surreal and funny and my hangover from the night before was kicking in, so I didn't give one shit.

"Get on here and try it out," I said. "You think it's firm enough?"

Camillus and the owner of the fine establishment that sold fresh-off-of-the-truck-slightly-damaged-but-almost-new wares looked at me and then each other, eyebrows raised with knowing.

"I think it's perfect, Sarah," he said. "I'll just take your word for it."

***

Two hours later, after he bought said mattress, sheets that wouldn't properly fit because the new mattress was not a standard size (which likely is why it *fell off the truck* in the first place), and a new coffee maker for the farm, Camillus and I sat across from each other at a little Mexican restaurant.

I don't remember what we ate.

I don't remember if anybody else was there.

I remember Camillus excused himself to go wash his hands before we ordered.

I remember I found this endearing and couldn't wait for him to get back to the table.

Oh no. Shit. I liked him.

We didn't talk about Mom, and we didn't talk about his divorce.

He asked me about my work at Adobe and if I liked living in San Francisco. He made eye contact with me the entire time. He was interested in what I had to say.

I suddenly felt like we were on a date.

But it wasn't a date.

Was this a date?

We drank Pacifico. He tilted the bottom of his bottle up in the air after he pushed in the lime wedge, and it made a popping sound when he removed his thumb, which made me laugh. I asked him to do the same with my beer.

Oh no.

OH NO.

OH NO.

I liked him.

***

The entire drive home I couldn't stop thinking about kissing him.

I already knew I might want to sleep with him to get my mind off Mom's cancer, but I didn't know how much I wanted to feel him kissing me until I spent the day with him.

I wanted to kiss Camillus Musselman, and I wanted him to kiss me.

He pulled in front of the house and carried in the coffee maker as I checked on Mom, who was asleep in the bedroom.

I walked out to the front room where he was standing, the door left open behind him, the space filled with what started to feel like awkward silence, like we both wondered how to say goodbye.

"Well, um, thanks for a fun day," I said.

"You're welcome," he said. "And thank you for helping me find a mattress, Sarah."

I loved that he said my name so often, as if he liked hearing himself say it. I was trying to read his expressions and remembered that Thanksgiving night down in the cave when I didn't yet know I liked him.

We awkwardly hugged with some football-player-like slaps on the back, the "I'm hugging you, but I'm not really hugging you" hugs men employ to remain manly.

I didn't care. Somehow, with the mix of the mattress buying, the two beers, the freckle on his nose I'd never noticed before, my desire to feel good about something, and my desire to see this man smile again, I decided to kiss him.

He pulled away.

He shook his head.

He raised both hands up and waved them around the way you do when you want something to stop, like he was disappointed, angry even.

I felt foolish, like a little kid who had done something wrong, and suddenly I feared I'd misread the fun of our nondate date and what felt like real chemistry.

He walked out the door, and I followed him to the driveway.

"It's supposed to be fun, Camillus!" I half shouted at the back of his head, hoping humor might make this not feel like rejection.

He stopped and turned around, looking back at me, still a little dumbfounded perhaps.

He didn't say a word.

But then he smiled. That smile. His smile.

Even though I wasn't at all sure what he thought of me, I liked Camillus Musselman.

DUCKS ON THE APPALACHIAN TRAIL

Therapy is not like hiking the Appalachian Trail. I mean, I've never hiked any part of the Appalachian Trail, so I'm not 100 percent positive, but my keen sense of perception tells me that you generally start at one point, hike until the next point, and so on and so forth until you arrive at the decided-upon destination for that leg of the hike. And then the next day, you repeat the process from a new starting point, moving in one direction, forward, until you reach your goal. I'm not saying it's easy, but you keep covering distance—you get there by putting one foot in front of the other. Then you can look back at the map and see markers of your progress, how far you've come, on a clear, measurable path.

That's not how therapy goes.

For me, therapy is like being a duck paddling around the same pond in seemingly random circles, over and over, hoping to find bugs or crumbs to eat along the way, diving down under the surface and coming back up, not sure where the shoreline is but aware that it must be there, because that's how you got into this pond in the first place. And you keep swimming around in circles, diving down and coming back up, finding small bites of nourishment, enough to keep going, but you can never really say what bug, what bread crumb, what particular morsel thrown in by some tourist was the one that filled you up. You just know you're being nourished, that this pond is giving you what you need to survive.

I'm not sure whether David is the bug, the tourist, or the pond, or whether this analogy even holds up, so please don't consult a duck expert. What I am saying is that therapy is *not* a straight path, that the progress is not marked by a sign telling you that you've arrived. Progress comes from making sense of the circles, seeing patterns in what you thought was random.

From our first session, I knew David would never just *tell me* what he thought was going on with me, even if he had a hunch. He needed me to arrive at things on my own, and he did this by asking me questions, questions that often pissed me off.

SCOTT KENNEDY, FOR EXAMPLE

"So you've said there's a voice in your head. What does it sound like?" David prompted.

"Well, it's me," I said after a minute of thinking. "I mean, it's my voice telling me how much I suck, how I'm not skinny enough, or successful enough, or smart enough, over and over. It's like a tape or film strip that keeps running from the time I wake up in the morning until I go to bed."

He nodded. "Is the tape running when you're at work?"

I almost laughed in response—it never stopped. "Oh, it's running all of the time in an endless loop," I said. "So even when I'm doing a presentation or leading a meeting, I have to try to quiet the voice on the tape and do the work I need to do. It's pretty exhausting, and I wonder what it would be like if it wasn't running. Imagine everything more I could do then. Just think about all of those gold stars I could get!"

I had told David about the gold-stars thing early on, and he knew how much I liked to achieve. As we got to know each other, I always tried to make him smile or laugh during every session, especially when I needed a little break.

He paused, considering. "Well, why don't we try to give the voice a name, because even if it's coming from you, it's really just a side of you, and it might be helpful to name it," he said.

"Like, a real name?" I asked. "What kind of name? Like Susannah or Percy or maybe Fleetwood Mac? How do I know what to call it?"

I was a little annoyed by this exercise because I wasn't yet comfortable with our seemingly random circles and didn't know to trust David's methods, and sometimes I wanted those handy mile markers of progress.

"Can you think of somebody you don't like, somebody who wronged you in some way? That could be a good way to give a name to the self-loathing for our purposes here."

"SCOTT KENNEDY!"

I shouted like a contestant on a quiz show. David looked surprised that I was so certain this could be the right name, but I knew it was.

Scott Kennedy. The red-headed boy from second grade at Chandlersville Elementary. He picked on me all of the time, teasing me and chasing me on the playground.

One spring day at recess, I was on the monkey bars and he kept pulling my legs from below. I asked him to stop. He did it again and I asked him to stop again. The third time, I jumped down, pushed him to the ground, and pinned his arms down the way my brother did when he tickled me, but instead of tickling, I punched him right in the face as hard as I could. I'd asked him to stop picking on me, and he just wouldn't listen. So I punched him again. Maybe three times. Mom had to come pick me up from the principal's office, and she could barely keep a straight face on the way home. She again had to stifle a laugh when she shared over dinner that the youngest Gormley was sent home from second grade for beating up Scott Kennedy by the monkey bars.

I hadn't thought about that kid for thirty years, and here we were, sitting in my therapist's office in Manhattan talking about Scott Kennedy. I was laughing so hard at the memory, I forgot we were supposed to be working on something important.

David smiled. "So how do you feel about Scott Kennedy—the voice, not the kid you beat up on the playground?"

"What do you mean, how do I feel about him?" I asked. "He's just always there, reminding me that I'm not good enough. I guess I've gotten used to it, and I'm still getting everything done in life. It's just—God, it's exhausting sometimes."

"Well," David prodded. "Do you think Scott Kennedy is right about you?"

I paused. "I don't know. I mean, yes," I answered. "I think he must be right even though I hate it—hate him—and wish the voice—sorry— that *he* would shut the fuck up and leave me alone."

"Why don't you stand up for yourself?" David asked. "Can you tell him to fuck off and leave you alone?"

It was a good question. "I don't know," I responded. "I've never tried, because I don't know what I would say. I guess I agree with him when he tells me I'm ugly and not smart enough, that I'll never really succeed, so I just try not to listen, but it's always there. And yes, I know that by most measures I'm doing okay, that I'm attractive and successful yadda yadda, but I just wish I could feel good about myself. Does that make sense?"

"Yes, that makes sense," David said, "but I think you're missing something by not standing up to him."

I sat there silently, wishing I could give David what he wanted but getting frustrated because I didn't know how to do what he was suggesting, didn't know how to feel something other than what I'd been feeling for so long. He saw my furrowed brow and after a few minutes suggested another method of understanding.

"So," he said. "We know what Scott Kennedy thinks of you. What about other people who know you—really know you?"

"You mean like work people?" I started. "They all think I'm great—smart, funny, successful Sarah, the one you want to be your boss and the one you want to have drinks with after work. But I don't think they count because they only see me at work."

"Well, who else might you trust?" he asked. "You've told me about your DePauw friends. Do you think they really know who you are? I want you to picture them walking into your apartment, how they would greet you, and how they might describe you."

I couldn't talk because the tears started coming fast, hot streaks burning down my face, snot starting to drip from my nose. There were no words to describe my friends to David, what they meant to me, the feeling that came over me when I started seeing their faces one at a time as they came into my fancy apartment on West Twenty-Third, the one my Martha Stewart salary helped pay for, with the big terrace and views over the High Line and the Hudson River. Brooks, then Nancy and Tippett, Shawna, Hegman, and Fran. Fran with her sweet smile and "Hi, Gorms," as she rounded out the crew. I could hear their voices, these friends of mine, my girls, and I could see them light up when they saw me, feel Brooks hugging me extra hard with one of her special squeezes at the end.

I was crying because David brought me there, right up to the place where I was going to have to acknowledge that the people who knew me best actually adored me. What I didn't know yet was that even if you understand something intellectually, it can take years to let yourself believe it and even longer to let yourself feel it.

AT A BAR NEAR THE AIRPORT

A few days after my nondate, mattress-buying outing with Camillus, I flew back to San Francisco to close that chapter of my life. I decided to put everything in storage and only take home the things I thought I might need for my grown-up gap year, which were really just clothes and my two bad cats.

As I went through jeans and sweaters—yes to the Levi's and gray cashmere V-neck, no to the too-tight black skirt—my mind kept going back to Camillus and how I wanted to talk to him again, even with all of the awful unknowns in my life. Then I thought about how hard and strange it must be for him to be going through so much change in *his* life.

I knew that rationally, us dating made no sense. My life was a mess. His life was a mess. There was so much at risk given how close he was to my brother, how often we might see each other given the small-town-ness of life in Ohio, and how awkward things would be if we dated and broke up, which was what I expected since that's how every relationship of mine for the past, well, *forever* had ended. And my original plan of some good-for-the-soul-but-bad-idea casual sex was now out of the question because I knew I liked him.

I called Nancy, as I did most days. She now lived in Shaker Heights with her husband and four kids. People sometimes think we are sisters given we both have shitty Irish skin, as we like to call it.

"Do I text Camillus again or just let it go?" I asked her.

"Well, do you want me to be honest or just tell you what you want to hear?" she said.

I laughed. We both knew I wanted her to tell me what I wanted to hear.

"Even if you go out a few times and it doesn't go anywhere, you're going to have to be mature about it so it's not awkward with Joe, so why not?" she said. "He sounds like a great guy, and trust me, if he just got divorced he is not going to want to get serious with anyone anytime soon. So, go drink a beer with him and have some fun."

I would land in Columbus Monday night around five and could see if he wanted to meet up again. Of course, he might already have plans or be busy with his kids—or just not want to see me at all. Even at forty-five, I was still just a girl who didn't want to be rejected, even by text.

But then I thought about his smile, how he had the slightest lisp when he said certain words, and how good I felt when he said my name. I sent the text.

"Hey there, I land tomorrow around five. Let me know if you want to grab a drink before I head to the farm."

Delivered.

Nothing.

Fifteen minutes.

Thirty minutes.

What was he doing? Was he calling a friend to ask what *he* should do?

I kept trying to busy myself and not obsess about his lack of a response. That's the deal. Once you put a text out there, you have to be prepared for whatever comes back, even if there's no reply at all, which is a singular and terrible form of misery.

And then the three magic dots on my iPhone appeared.

***

Dark gray cashmere sweater. Light gray cashmere scarf. Levi's. Black loafers. My winter travel uniform was now a date outfit, even though I wasn't sure if this was a date.

I left the parking garage and walked into what looked like a sports bar to meet him. I wondered how I would look to him. My hair was pulled back the last time I saw him, and now my mop of blond curls fell around my shoulders, handy for nervous hair twisting. I had stopped in the ladies' room after the long flight from San Francisco to put on some makeup, entirely aware of how little difference it would make. But I wanted him to think I was pretty.

And then I saw him look up from the bar. He'd shaved his beard and looked even more handsome in a checked dress shirt, jeans, and a blue Patagonia zip-front vest. I guessed that it might be his uniform. Broad shoulders, strong arms. His hands. His wrists. I could feel my heart racing, knew I was blushing, and hoped he didn't notice.

"Oh hi, Sarah." He lingered on my name the same way he had on the mattress-buying trip. Looking at me in a way that said, "I know what your name is and you know I know what your name is, but I'm going to keep saying *Sarah*."

"Oh hi, Camillus."

I already liked saying his name too. He got up and gave me a hug. The structure of him calmed me. He was solid. A man. Shit, I liked him.

I don't recall what we talked about, but I imagine some stuff about San Francisco, my packing, his divorce, whether there was anything new happening with Mom, and whether the burger or the chicken sandwich was better. An hour or so passed. I wanted to sit there all night but needed to get home to Mom.

He asked for the check.

There was a long pause in the conversation.

I looked at him, trying to read him, but knew I had to ask the question we'd both been trying to answer for ourselves.

"So what do you think we should do?"

I stopped myself from saying more, from saying all of the reasons we shouldn't date, which I knew he already knew. He took a drink of his Miller Lite, put the bottle down, and then turned toward me on his barstool.

"Well, Sarah, I think we should give it a shot."

I stammered for a second and tried to conceal the smile spreading across my face.

"Oh, well, good, um, great, yes." I got words out to fill the air as I processed. "I mean, I think we should, too, and I'm so happy you think so."

In the next minute, as he signed the check and then went to the men's room, I sat there flabbergasted. This was the first time in my life that I sat with a man as we decided together that, yes, we would try something. With words in conversation rather than trying to decode another messy sexual episode in a blurry bedroom. Despite the long list of reasons not to, despite the mess of our individual lives, we would give it a shot. We would take the risk you have to take when you want to see what might happen.

I grabbed his hand as we walked to the garage, and he chuckled to himself but loud enough that I could hear.

"Look at us, holding hands," he said. "I'm holding hands with Sarah Gormley."

He kissed me and I kissed him back. Sweet and slow and hard and fast. Teasing, tasting, darting tongues and hungry hands devouring everything we could before we pulled apart and laughed at ourselves because we were two fortysomethings making out in a parking garage at a mall in Ohio.

DATING

I was forty-five the day Camillus and I decided to try something. Forty-five, and the longest I'd really ever dated anyone as an adult was three months, maybe longer if you include the breakups and getting-back-together bullshit. I didn't know much except that I wasn't good at dating if dating "success" meant a relationship, which I thought it did. I either chose the wrong men or didn't like the right ones, or some blurry mix of both wrongs. So many wrongs.

I did learn this along the way: if you've never had a healthy romantic relationship, it's pretty fucking hard to recognize when you're in one that's, well, *not* healthy.

Sure, you know how to date and play the game with your friends, asking why he didn't call, and will he call, and is this the one, and does he really care about you or is he stressed at work—that must be it—and who wouldn't want to go out with you. Then you go get another bottle of wine. That part of dating I mastered all the way back in my early twenties, inspired by a beautiful Nigerian man who told me I looked better in Levi's 501 jeans than any man or woman he'd ever met. He also told me a story about how as a little boy growing up in Nigeria, he was afraid oranges were going to grow in his stomach when he accidentally swallowed the seeds, and I convinced myself that this revelation and sweet vulnerability made us a perfect match. Never mind that he was unreliable, had a girlfriend who sometimes called at 2 a.m. when I stayed over, and quite possibly fucked every attractive person in Chicago.

But that's not the point.

The point is that if I had the time to write you the whole story of my useless romantic endeavors, including every specific detail, you would be so mad at me, our love-challenged, curly-haired heroine, by the end that you might actually throw the book across the room. I was dumb, dumb, dumb. And I'm not dumb. I had all of those scorecards to prove it. And still, I kept choosing men whose *only* common denominator was that they weren't good for me.

David later helped me understand the "Velcro effect," which means that you pick partners who match or enhance the way you already feel about yourself, so I was kind of fucked on that front. When you already feel like shit about yourself, you choose people who help you keep feeling like shit. Now that we're older and wiser, we can see this pattern, but then? No way could I see it. It was going to take years for me to undo that behavior.

The worst, most painful one was the married guy. Smart and funny, he reminded me of my dad in the best way—not the I'm-secretly-in-love-with-Dad way, I promise. I made fun of how he wore his reading glasses like an old man. He made fun of me for coming into the office with wet hair, and I explained how curls need to air dry. He told me how much he liked it when he smelled my Trish McEvoy No. 3 and knew he had taken the same elevator as me that morning.

Our formula was ripe for a disastrous ending given that his married-guy attitude permitted him to convince himself there was nothing wrong with texting me first thing in the morning and last thing at night because we weren't hooking up. Hints of intimacy without real intimacy. Not hooking up? Not an affair. Simple, right?

I was so mired in disbelief that any man would find me truly attractive that I didn't realize any real feelings were there—what women's magazines love to call an emotional affair, which can be *far more* damaging and painful than sexual infidelity, if you're taking notes from the magazines—until I was thinking about him all of the time, awaiting the texts, hoping for lunch or time for a drink after work. We kissed only once, and it was powerful enough that he stopped texting me and started going to therapy. I eventually got another big job and tried to recover from the loss of him. In hindsight, I can see that we did have a real connection and friendship, possibly some form of love. But not once along the way did any internal alarm sound suggesting he wasn't the right guy for me, that this wasn't the right kind of love because he was *married.*

I wish I could tell you that one was the wake-up call. But there were more.

There was the one who told me to meet him at a restaurant that had two different locations, and when I asked which one, he told me to figure it out. I kept dating him. I dated him for three more months, cried about the breakup as if there was an actual loss, and then tried to get *back together* with him. There was the one who forgot to tell me he had a DUI, so I had to do all of the driving when we went down to the shore to see the family compound he liked to brag about, the compound he didn't have keys to because the family didn't trust him. Even after my father said to me, "You know, Sarah, you don't have to bring them *all* home," I still took that one home to the farm for Thanksgiving.

Another one invited me to a wedding in Miami. Nice, right? I bought my own ticket, and he sat in first class and left me in coach, looking up the aisle at his half profile, leaning over an armrest through that weird sheer curtain that divides the classes in more ways than one. The entire flight down I thought about what to say once we arrived— thought about booking a return flight back to New York right then. But I didn't book the return flight. I didn't tell him "Go fuck yourself," or "Good luck finding somebody else dumb enough to put up with this bullshit," because I so desperately wanted to be loved.

I can now see that I wanted these men to provide something I hadn't even done for myself: to appreciate who I was, to treat me with kindness, as somebody special who deserved to be loved, adored even. When you ache for something unknown, it's easy to get confused about the actual experience you're in.

When I finally found a good man, I broke up with him. He was kind, smart, thoughtful, and sensitive, with a body so beautiful it still kind of makes me mad just thinking about it. He didn't work out or diet, yet it was as if Michelangelo sketched him every night, making more improvements just to tease me. His big flaw? He liked me *too* much. He called when he said he would, showed up just because he wanted to kiss me, and checked in on me with saltines and 7Up when I didn't feel well. I didn't know what to do with such a foreign feeling, with what I believed to be his profound kindness and goodness. I didn't know how to receive love and didn't yet know that people can be kind to themselves *and* other people too.

We took a trip to Big Sur with friends of his and rented a cabin for the night before heading back to San Francisco. The place was faux roughing it for city types, and there was a flock of wild turkeys that were actually quite tame roaming around the grounds. I looked out at him one morning after breakfast as he smoked his Marlboro on the front porch, this gorgeous six-foot-four-inch human being who would do anything for me. A turkey approached and instead of shooing it away or ignoring the damn thing, he cowered, crouching down and then flailing his arms in fear, cigarette still lit. I decided right then that this was not my man, not him, not this guy afraid of tame wild turkeys, not this guy who loved me, believed in me, even adored me. Him? Not a chance.

I broke up with him the next night. On New Year's Eve, no less.

WHAT STORY IS THIS?

You might be wondering why I'm telling you about my dating history and this man named Camillus. You may have thought you were reading a story about Mom and me coming home to the farm to be with her—how I finally started healing as she was dying.

That was supposed to be the order; it felt destined to be the order that day I drove up the driveway when we knew her cancer was back. That could be the whole story, but then, whammo, this man named Camillus showed up. In what world? In whose movie script does this happen? Cue up the Hallmark marathon and put on your fuzzy slippers.

When we look back at things, we imply an order, and the minute the words go down on the page, the thing already happened. A moment passed, a memory recalled. How we felt then versus how we feel now and what matters to the story. I want to make sense of these things.

From the day we shopped for mattresses until now, even as I'm typing these words knowing they are already past tense, I'm still trying to assign the right series of words to this man named Camillus. I am still surprised by this love.

CHEMO SHIT

Watching a parent go through cancer makes you the most rational crazy person you'll ever meet. On the one hand, you are calm and comforting—you're the caregiver, after all, and you are rational because *somebody* needs to be. On the other hand, you spend more energy on little things like whether her washcloth is clean and whether the remote control is in the exact right spot for her to reach because the big thing that is happening is unfathomable.

The nurse talked into the little device clipped to her scrubs near her collarbone. She looked young to me—too young to have a job in the cancer center we visited weekly for chemo. She looked like she should be wearing cutoff jean shorts and flip-flops and drinking beer in some dive bar and not trying to help people stay alive by feeding poison into their frail bodies.

"I need help pushing at Station Four," I heard her say.

Did she say *"pushing"*? I wasn't positive, but any time I'd heard anyone use that word in a hospital setting in a movie or on a TV show, it meant somebody was having a baby. And nobody was having a baby around this place as far as I could tell. Mom and I looked at each other and stayed quiet, assuming that Too-Young Nurse knew what she was doing.

Another nurse who seemed more experienced, with visible wisps of gray hair, came into the curtained-off station, and we helped Mom stand up to lean onto the table. As part of her treatment, they were giving her shots, two of them, one in each of her tiny little butt cheeks, the sight of which would have made me gasp except I didn't want to remind Mom of what she already knew: her body was disappearing.

They called it "pushing" because the clear, viscous liquid didn't squirt out from a syringe like you imagine it would when they're testing it. This was something far different, something more like a gel. I couldn't believe they were pushing this stuff into Mom. She made a quick yelping noise indicating she was in pain, and I suddenly wanted to hit the younger nurse and grab the big plastic syringe and shoot the thick, gooey substance into her ass. I was so mad at her for hurting Mom and for being young and healthy, even though I knew she was just doing her job and trying to help Mom stay alive when she could have been anywhere else doing anything else at that moment.

***

I was obsessed with Mom eating. And yes, I recognize the irony given our tangled dance of striving to be skinny by not eating. But this wasn't the time for some big aha moment or an essay about inherited disorders. This was about trying to help a dying woman be a healthier version of a dying woman. How's that for some fucked-up logic?

She didn't want to eat and told me nothing tasted good. Every morning I would offer her coffee and toast or a yogurt, and every morning she would tell me she wasn't hungry. Some mornings she would placate me and try to eat the toast or half a banana, which often led to her vomiting into the white porcelain dish with the blue flowers she loved so much because it was the perfect size for warming up leftover succotash in the summer. She would throw up mostly brown liquid, and then I would hand her a towel to wipe her mouth and take the dish into the bathroom to flush away the vomit while simultaneously trying to keep my dry heaves from turning into my own puking.

I still wanted her to eat, though.

Food meant calories, which meant energy, which meant there might be a chance, or something close to a chance, of keeping her alive. I didn't know what else to do except urge her to eat, to try to eat.

***

Mom looked at me from her chair in the front room one morning and cleared her throat a bit, letting me know she was going to say something. Jane had stopped by to say hello before she went to work, and Joe had been there to drop off the paper, checking in as he did every morning. We developed a rhythm that kept the days moving, even as they all started to blend together as the treatment continued and we tried to pretend like Mom might get better.

She put down her crossword puzzle and pulled her glasses down to the end of her nose.

"Do you think we should write my obituary today?"

I gave her the two raised eyebrows with wide-open eyes.

"Uhmm," I started. "No, I do not think we need to write your obituary today. I think that might be just a little premature, considering you're doing a crossword puzzle and you told me you're actually hungry for the first time in weeks. Why don't we go get breakfast and not write your obituary, if that's okay with you?"

She smiled and nodded.

We drove to a greasy spoon about ten minutes away from the farm, where Mom ordered everything on the menu the way a little kid might if it was their sixth birthday: scrambled eggs, a biscuit, a side of bacon, orange juice, and a waffle with strawberries and whipped cream.

I was so happy I sent Jane and Joe a photo of Mom with her personal breakfast buffet spread out in front of her.

She told me the whipped cream tasted so good that she thought her appetite must really be coming back. As I paid the check, I thought about making some real whipped cream to have in the fridge in case she might want more later in the day or even the next morning.

ACTUAL SHIT

About three minutes into the drive home, I heard the distinct gurgle of a very unhappy stomach. It occurred to me then that she had just consumed about six times the amount of food she had eaten in the previous week, which probably wasn't the best thing for her already-delicate system.

"I'm going to need to get to a bathroom somewhere immediately," she said.

"We'll be home in, like, five minutes," I replied, gripping the wheel. "Just hold on."

I thought about alternative routes home—if I had taken Spry Road, would that have been faster? I knew I had to get her to a bathroom as soon as possible, and I could tell she was struggling.

"I'm not sure I can make it," she said.

I thought about where we could stop. The McCutcheon farm was coming up on the left, and I knew they wouldn't mind, but then Mom would have to answer all sorts of questions about her cancer and treatment, which she would *not* want to do.

"Stop at McCutcheons'?" I half-heartedly suggested. "It'll be four more minutes after that."

"NO!" came her response. "Drive faster."

I flashed back to one summer when we were on our way to a family reunion. I was driving and Mom was in the passenger seat with her famous baked beans on the floor at her feet. At some point, I took a corner too fast, and some of the beans spilled over and she yelled at me: "Jesus, Sarah, what are you trying to do here? DRIVE FLAT. DRIVE FLAT, dammit!" I burst into laughter and told her that her comment made no sense, that there's no such thing as "driving flat," and that maybe she should calm down and stop yelling at me. We laughed the rest of the way to the reunion.

Now I was driving as fast as I could down Clay Pike without being too reckless because I didn't think killing both of us in a car accident seemed like a good idea, especially as our obituaries weren't written yet.

We flew past Fullers golf course, down the hill, and over the little bridge. I was happy Clay Pike wasn't a gravel road anymore, the way it was most of my childhood—when you hit the gravel at a certain speed, you would fishtail and end up in the ditch in no time.

"Hold on, hold on," I said. "We are going to be home in like two minutes."

I looked over at her and she was totally quiet, and then her face told me what I already knew before she said it aloud.

"It doesn't matter now," she said.

Less than two miles from the house, Mom shit in her pants right there in the truck. I felt horribly for her and felt slightly sorry for myself, but then I laughed. The hard, guttural laughs that can save you from crying sometimes. And then she started laughing at me and with me and then we repeated what she said together, the line that would become a new part of our regular repartee.

"It doesn't matter now."

The shitting the pants didn't matter, but the moment did. As I watched her get out of the truck and head into the house, trying to walk normally—which for her wasn't even possible on a good day thanks to the steel rods from her back surgery years before, much less than when she has just shit her pants—I loved her as much as I could ever recall loving her. I wanted her to stay alive as long as possible. Not because I needed her, but because I wanted her in my life and wanted to keep getting to know her, even on a morning like this one.

SYMMETRY

SUSAN CAMERON GORMLEY

SARAH CAMERON GORMLEY

Look at our names.

The symmetry, the *S-C-G*, the seven syllables unfolding across the page, two-three-two, like a short haiku, one created exclusively for Mom and me.

Better yet, say the names aloud, slowly. The soft *S* that slides over the tongue, then the hard *C* of *Cam-e-ron*. The graceful *G* and the denouement of *ley*, letting you know you've come to the end of something.

Some girls obsessively wrote boys' names in the margins of their notebooks, believing that if they wrote their names enough times, the fantasy relationships would come true.

Not me.

I wrote my own name, again and again, enthralled by the flow of the pen on the page, each letter a reminder that I was lucky to be my parents' daughter. I was so lucky, in fact, that I had *both* of their names in mine.

Sarah came from Grandpa Cameron's mother. They decided to give me *Cameron* because it became Mom's middle name once she married Dad.

As a third grader, I assumed that I, too, would get married one day. My plan was to start using Sarah C. G. Newlastname to retain all the parts of me, just like Mom. I wanted to be like her in every way and didn't yet know what I was really hoping for and how different we might truly be.

***

Everyone loved Susan Gormley.

They wanted to be like her. They wished they could walk into a room the way she did, head held high with short silver—and later in life, white—hair, accessorized with nothing more than a simple gold wedding band and a dab of Chanel No. 5 on each wrist and on her collarbone for special occasions.

Her beauty was the thing. And her beauty was her attitude.

Everyone wanted to be like Mom because she was smart, had ideas, told you what she thought, and didn't give a rat's ass who you were—if you were acting like an asshole, Susan Gormley told you so. "You know what, Wilson? Shut the fuck up. You're lucky she married your dumb ass in the first place, so cool it. And pass the potatoes." That was for Dr. Wilson, who liked to pick on his wife, Carol, once he had his second Crown Royal. Carol was quiet and sweet, two words never assigned to Mom, and that was part of her charming ire. She didn't like mean people. Couldn't stand bullies. And guess what? Dr. Wilson didn't even blink. He shut up and passed the potatoes, and the conversation picked back up around the table. I would watch her as a little girl and think, *Mom is a woman who has it all figured out.*

Friends confided that they wished she could be *their* mother because they felt like she believed in them and really understood them more than their own moms. I knew she was sharing her light with them, and somehow I feared there wouldn't be enough left for me.

And if there wasn't, how would I grow up to be like her?

After years of therapy on my own, I could start to see Mom for who she was rather than the myth that grew around her. She was real. And complicated. A woman who could be infuriatingly judgmental when she didn't approve and infinitely kind if she thought you didn't have somebody rooting for you. A mother who admitted to me over drinks at a spa that she wasn't always sure she should be a mother. A wife who got jealous when Dad flirted with women at the club. A dutiful daughter to her own mother, who never told her she loved her.

Mom was so much more than her myth.

NAPTIME

Mom was a woman who napped.

Everyone knew this about her. Susan Gormley cussed, drove too fast, and took naps. "My bed is calling" was her line when she was weary or just needed a little break. Her naps meant that I napped, even when I felt too old for such things. I spent lots of time sitting at the top of the stairway waiting for her to get up from her naps. I would agree to nap in my room, pretend to get into my bed, and then sit at the top of the steps waiting to hear her stir so we could figure out what we would do next with our day.

In the summer we would go out to one of the gardens, and I would help her water the boxwoods, moving the slowly trickling hose when she told me it was time. Or we would weed, making a pile to be thrown over the fence into the field when we finished. We might go down to Salt Creek to look for tadpoles and pick wildflowers. She taught me about the bright red Indian paintbrush and black-eyed Susans, which I thought were named after her.

On many days, I would simply climb up on Dad's side of the bed and sit next to her. We would talk as we waited for Jane and Joe to get off the bus and come up the driveway, and I could feel her really listening to me. Even though I knew Dad was her number one, Mom was my favorite. We became pals in a way that felt like our secret. Our friendship started there, in that bed, just the two of us.

Looking back, I can see that Mom's naps and regular need to escape to her bed were part of something else going on with her, but I didn't know what until years later.

DR. PORTER—SCENE 1

I never would have imagined that Mom was depressed if she hadn't been sitting in front of me telling me that she was.

Shortly after I graduated from college, we were having a glass of wine at Bistro 110, a restaurant in Chicago. Mom recalled the appointment she made with a therapist in Columbus ten years prior when she was worried about Dad being depressed. I had observed his red Corvette and his penchant for ordering expensive suits from his personal shopper at Ralph Lauren in New York and figured it was a run-of-the-mill midlife crisis.

"Dr. Porter first talked to us together and then met with each of us individually," she explained. "I was so worried about how it was going to go with your dad."

I always loved watching Mom talk because she used her hands, with the palm of her hand close to her face and her fingers cupping at something, probably an idea she was holding for you to understand, the gestures somehow making her opinions bigger.

"Well, wouldn't you know it, after he met with us one-on-one, the three of us sat down together again and he told us he thought Dad was fine, that he didn't seem depressed at all. Then he turned to *me* and said that he suspected *that I was the one who was depressed*!"

She laughed as she told me this, not in a this-is-absurd way, but more of an aha way. It's telling that Mom hadn't protested his assessment and agreed to go back for another appointment. Not Susan-Gormley-like at all, and a sign of just how much she was hurting. Mom admitted that she had never known what she was feeling or what to call it, just that she felt bad.

"I can look back and see that I was struggling in my late twenties and thirties but never thought it could be depression because what in the hell did I have to be depressed about?"

Mom also said she didn't think she had the stamina for talk therapy. "My friend Jean told me therapy was the hardest thing she's ever done, and I just didn't want to dig into all of that crap. I wanted to feel better."

I don't know how many more times Mom met with him, but Dr. Porter prescribed Prozac, which became a part of her daily routine.

Looking back now, I can see her *need* to tell me. It was because she trusted me but also, somehow, wanted my approval as her friend. We were so close, and we depended on each other in a way that was beautiful, something my friends and other mothers admitted they envied. Our relationship was special, something important in my life, something that defined me, and Mom.

I was happy that Mom confided in me, and hated that she had been in pain for so much of her life. I couldn't yet recognize that emotional suffering might be something we shared—one of our common denominators like our initials, blue eyes, and high arches. I wonder if she understood or felt guilty about the possibility that I might be depressed too.

After all, she took me to see Dr. Porter when she realized that I might be anorexic.

DR. PORTER—SCENE 2

One Friday night my senior year, Mom decided I was *too* skinny. I planned to pick up my friend Christy and go to the boys' varsity basketball game down at Morgan High School. I was wearing jeans, a light blue button-down blouse, and brown leather boots. My belt was too big, even on the last hole, so I figured out how to wrap it around and tuck it in under the second loop. I looked cute and planned to leave before Mom and Dad ate dinner, knowing I wouldn't want to add calories to the day. I told them I would eat popcorn at the game. When I got to the bottom of the stairs, Mom looked up and kind of gasped at me.

"What?" I asked, thinking it was something about my outfit. "Do I not look okay for the game? I love this shirt, and you bought it for me."

"No, honey," she said. "It's your hip bones. They're poking out."

"No, they're not. The jeans are just stretched out because I haven't washed them in a while."

Even though I hoped to explain away the flimsy denim, I knew something had shifted, that Mom wasn't going to let it go, and I tried to gauge whether her look was anger or concern by the way her head was tilted, her hands on her own slender hips.

"Sarah, come in here with me," she said. She took me by the hand and walked me into her bathroom, where we stood side by side in front of the full-length mirror.

I looked at our reflections.

"What? What, Mom?" I asked.

She turned toward me, put her hands on my shoulders, and looked me in the eye. "Do you not see it, honey? How are you not seeing this?"

"What are you talking about?"

"Sarah, you are too fucking skinny. You have to start eating more."

My immediate reaction was fear—a sudden horrible image of me having to eat plate after plate of cheesy lasagna in front of them, the inevitable weight gain, the undoing of all of my work. But then I took a breath and settled into myself. I calmly told her what she wanted to hear—that she was right, maybe I had lost a little weight, and I would make sure to remember to eat more. I let her off the hook with my goodness. At the same time, all in that same half of a minute, framed like a still life, I felt a little sting of pride, because I knew I was still winning this game.

I was so skinny that Mom finally noticed, but I also knew I could keep going.

The next week we drove to Columbus to meet with Dr. Porter. I had no idea she already knew him, as Mom was not yet willing to share with me that she was taking Prozac every day per his recommendation. I was nervous on the hourlong drive, and we didn't talk much except for Mom saying that she was glad we were doing this, that she was worried about me, and that he might be able to help.

"I don't need help, really, I promise," I told her, keenly aware that I shouldn't protest too much, that I had to find the balance that would allow her to feel better.

I recall very little about the room or even where I sat. I remember Dr. Porter had glasses and reminded me of the actor Tony Randall from *The Odd Couple*.

"Sarah, it's nice to meet you. As you know, your mom is concerned about you. So why don't we start with you telling me how you're feeling and whether you believe you have something going on with food and eating."

My nerves shifted. Something in his posture told me I would be able to outsmart this man, that this would be easy. Even though he was a doctor, he was just a box checker. He didn't want to deal with my mess. I was a really good anorexic, and I was really good at telling people the story they wanted to believe—that I was perfectly fine. Nobody *wants* to believe that any kid has a problem, especially not the good kids. I knew how to play the part.

"I know why Mom is concerned," I insisted, with the right tone of apology mixed with certainty. "I know I'm thin, but I am not sick. I burn almost 1,200 calories in a single basketball practice. There's no way I could get through varsity practices if I'm not eating enough to fuel my body."

I promised him I knew how damaging anorexia could be to a girl's health and that I'd never do that to myself or to Mom and Dad. Once I could tell he was really listening, after I made him laugh about the disgusting food in the cafeteria, I looked him right in the eye and told him something I felt would close our deal.

"Eating disorders are just not that interesting—they are so cliché—and I'd never let myself be one of *those* girls."

I assured Dr. Porter that I was far too smart to have an eating disorder.

I permitted myself to enjoy moments that felt like small victories. I was so wrapped up in the story I was creating for others that I let myself feel good about the character I became. And I was so good at playing her that the other me—the real me, a young woman who was sad and hurting, with no idea why or what to do or where to turn—didn't stand a chance to develop, grow up, or get to know herself.

When you create a version of yourself and that version becomes who you are, how and when do you ever figure out who you were meant to be? These are the things I have been figuring out with David for ten years and am continuing to figure out, the types of things I wish Mom had talked about with Dr. Porter. We were both in pain. We both presented versions of ourselves to the world. Similar but not the same.

A WORD FROM AN ART GALLERY

I own an art gallery, but you don't need to hear about that yet. We'll get to that part. What you need to know now is that I'm sitting in an art gallery with my name on the door, writing about Mom. I have to get this part cleared up before I show you what happened at the farm in those last weeks and days. I'm trying to be honest, to tell you the truth about a woman who died, whose thin, pale hands I can still picture, whose blue eyes lit up every time she looked at me.

Like most of us, I had only one mother. Susan Gormley. Mom. She wanted things for me and for my siblings. She wanted us to be happy and to experience love, certainly. What mother doesn't want those things for her kids? But now, looking back and trying to make sense of things, I see how something was slightly off between us. From our afternoons of bagels and *Another World*, to the daily calls that continued until I moved home and we didn't need the phone anymore, Mom and I were always more like friends than a mother and a daughter. We absolutely relied upon each other, confided in each other, and, yes, loved the shit out of each other, but now I see I didn't always get what I needed.

The love between a mother and daughter is no tidy thing.

Unconditional love is a term I struggle with, because in my brain there was no such thing. And that intellectual certainty crept into my heart and lodged in there tight. How absurd is it to think anyone deserves love just for existing? That's something I never felt as a little girl or as a fully formed former little girl, frustrated by the way I was walking through the world, wanting things like love because I thought I earned them by doing, not by being. I was smart and skinny and successful, so *love me*, dammit. Somebody please fucking love me. I thought I had to earn love by accomplishing things rather than be loved simply because I woke up in the morning with a face full of freckles and my own blue eyes.

What if she had loved me differently? What if I had not deduced by age five that I could do certain things to make my parents happy? What came first? What is the order? Who can we blame for my self-loathing? How did Mom not see my pain? Why didn't she do something when I was little and obsessed with grades and test scores? Why couldn't she get out of her own way to be the mother I needed so I could become the real Sarah rather than the version of Sarah who hated herself for so long? I don't know, not entirely, and never will. Not with certainty. I can speculate and try to connect the dots, but mainly I can show you how I felt and how my perspective about her changed. I believe that she loved me the best way she could but that she had limitations. I believe Mom was in her own pain and perhaps didn't quite know how to love herself, which probably made being a mom pretty fucking hard sometimes.

Is it weird to wish for something different for your dead mother? Especially when you grew up wanting to be just like her? Mom was in pain and didn't know her pain could be fixed. I was in pain and didn't know my pain could be fixed. She medicated her pain away. The Prozac helped her suffer less. I therapied my pain away. The therapy helped me suffer less.

I don't want a trophy for doing the work. The trophy is finally liking myself and the way I show up in the world.

My sadness for Mom is that I'm not sure she ever felt the same thing.

DR. PORTER—SCENE 3

I received the message through my gallery's Facebook page in the summer of 2021. Columbus is a small city, and he's now retired and a portrait photographer, so it wasn't entirely surprising that he'd been following my art gallery since it opened.

"Are you Joe and Susan Gormley's daughter by chance?"

It was him. Dr. Porter. I could tell from his references to my parents that he had no idea that he had ever met me, which I found perplexing. But given that nearly thirty years had passed, I decided to forgive him.

Through a series of messages, we agreed to have a glass of wine on his patio overlooking downtown to talk about his art and likely much more. I was nervous, not dissimilar to how I'd felt on first dates, except this date was the man who prescribed antidepressants to my mom and, oh, by the way, overlooked the fact that I was starving myself. What does one wear to this "date" on a summer day in Ohio? The answer was a white linen shirt, green canvas pants, and strappy leather sandals.

We hugged hello. An awkward hug. Not sexual. More like how you might hug a distant cousin you haven't seen since childhood, but with the knowledge that you share some important history.

He was slight, with small black glasses that said, *I am smart, probably smarter than you.* I wanted to dislike him, but then he told me about his grandchildren as he prepared a cheese plate with more options than I thought the occasion warranted. He was a divorced grandfather who played the saxophone and loved taking photos of jazz musicians and mountain ranges.

"I admired and loved what little I knew about your parents and was so sorry to learn of their passing." As I was about to point out that he didn't really meet with them more than a handful of times—just once, for Dad—he filled in the blank.

"I didn't know them well, but sometimes you meet patients just once and never forget them. Your parents were like that. Great senses of humor, and I could tell they really loved each other."

My body reacted the way it still does when people say nice things about them: I got a little flushed, and the tears and snot started. After a few more niceties, I decided to remind him that he'd seen me. Not to scold him, but because I felt like this was a rare opportunity to close a loop.

"You probably don't remember, but I met with you once when I was a senior in high school. I had some eating stuff but did a really good job of covering it up, and you told Mom I was fine."

"My goodness, I'm sorry but I don't recall. You certainly seem healthy today."

Again, I thought I might be pissed off or want to yell at him for assuming anyone was fine based on a mere up and down, but that's not how I reacted. I simply wanted to tell him a little about my story.

"My eating stuff was really a symptom of something else. I had a whole bunch of self-loathing going on for most of my life and didn't begin to realize it until I started therapy when I was forty. It's been such a help, and I always wonder if Mom could have benefited from talk therapy as well. I know she didn't want to do it, so I guess we'll never know."

The air on his patio felt thick. I could tell he thought I was accusing him of something.

"Listen, Sarah—antidepressants are lifesavers for so many people, and there's no shame in using the right medication to help. Your mom was very clear that she had no interest in meeting regularly to talk about what was going on with her."

I nodded and agreed with him. "Oh yes, I know that—she told me."

And then he added something else that did bother me. This man who didn't know me but thought he did after one glass of Vermentino and small bites of cheese.

"I'll tell you another thing. There is no reason for you to ever be in pain like that again, and if you find yourself hurting, I can prescribe something or recommend another doctor who can. The meds work and you should take them."

The word "should" rubbed me the wrong way. I opened my mouth to defend myself because I hated him for a split second. My mom's psychiatrist. The man who missed my eating disorder. Right here in front of me—that has to be something *big*. Tell him he's wrong, Sarah—demand that he appreciate all of the work you've done with David and how you've changed your life.

But then I paused. I went inside of myself and realized I didn't need anything from this man. Relief came over me as I let go of the significance I thought this moment should hold. I leaned back in the metal bistro chair, looked out at the Scioto River, and reminded myself that he didn't know me and never would. What was important was what I thought about myself. I had brought myself out of the grips of anorexia in my early twenties by slowly and steadily choosing something better for myself. I was lucky I could do so. Then, still in pain in my forties, I navigated myself to therapy. I'd fought hard for myself. He was simply a doctor who had helped Mom, and the small world of Columbus, Ohio, brought us together on a warm summer night.

"Thank you, I'm good," I said in response to the suggestion of medication.

We exchanged pleasant goodbyes and hinted that we would do this again sometime, even though we both knew we weren't going to be friends.

A KNOT VERSUS A BOW

Untangling myself from Mom is something I will keep doing for the rest of my life.

I'd spent so long blaming myself and turning my anger inward that I had no time left to fault anyone else. And when it came to Mom and Dad, even trying to understand them in a new way felt too close to blame. David could see my struggle and navigated our conversation toward something useful. He progressively helped me see how much I idealized my parents, and asked questions about who they were and how they grew up so that I might see them in a new way—yes, as parents who loved me, but also as individuals who had their own distinct set of emotions and challenges that influenced their behavior.

We talked about how Mom doted on others and about how I felt watching her, always admiring her but also hurting because I felt she was giving away to others what should have been mine. I had worked so diligently to be what I thought she wanted me to be. And yet, there she was, seemingly passing out her love like cotton candy to people who were, in some cases, overweight, less educated, and even unable to keep a steady job, which was shocking to somebody like me, as I had convinced myself that I had to be skinny, smart, and successful to earn her love. If I was anything but perfect, I didn't believe I'd be worthy of her love.

"Why do you think she seemed to adore other people so easily, as you recall it?" he asked me once in his office in New York. I was crying less often six months in, but certain questions still got to me.

"I think she liked what she got in return, so it wasn't completely altruistic. I mean, I know it made her feel good in a weird way that people liked her as much or more than their own mothers."

"Do you have any idea why, though? Why did it seem to you that she was better at showing this kind of love to others than to her own children?"

Oh boy, that's when the tears started.

I flashed back to so many nights around the dining table when I watched her, always issuing the perfect insight, words of counsel laced with her trademark fucks and goddamns that never sounded crass but punctuated the air and made everyone feel at ease no matter the gravity of the topic. But maybe she performed on this stage not just because she felt good about herself but because that's where she felt better about herself than in any private moments with me, Jane, or Joe.

David filled in what I was reluctant to admit.

"Do you think maybe she didn't think she was a very good mother? Maybe she poured herself into other relationships that weren't as difficult for her? With others, she got to be this amazing, charismatic woman and could feel their affection in return, but the connection was safer because it was less close."

I'd never seen her in this light before. I'd never thought through just how hard on herself Mom might have been. If she thought she was a bad mother, she may have held herself back because she thought she would end up damaging us.

I nodded at David, picking up his hypothesis and what I was finally understanding.

"Maybe those relationships were easier for her because she wasn't filled with doubt and never had to be quite as vulnerable as she would have been with us, her own kids?" I wondered out loud. "Was it harder for her to be as loving to us because she doubted herself?"

I was cautious this time, posing thoughts as questions because it felt so odd to speculate about Mom in this way. But I knew I was on to something, and that happens in therapy sometimes. You say something aloud for the first time when the thought has been forming in you for years, lying fallow until the idea is ready to break the surface into the meaning you're finally willing to admit.

"I'd say that's entirely possible, Sarah," he said. "In fact, I'd think it's probable based on how you've described her."

I was so heavy with sadness for her suddenly, thinking about Grandma Cameron never telling Mom that she loved her, thinking about her trying so hard to be a good daughter and to make her parents proud, and then trying even harder to be a good wife and a good mom, to be what she thought other people wanted from her. And what if—despite all of those people telling her that she was one of the greats, one of their favorite people in the world—she still never felt good enough because the feeling wasn't coming from within her?

At that moment, I saw us as the same person, both of us contorting ourselves to try to be perfect, to be good enough, and to give people what they wanted from us.

I couldn't stop crying, wondering if she spent her whole life feeling as awful as I did. I could only imagine such pain was even possible because I was living it too.

I suddenly could see that maybe I took on Mom's pain as my own, which is something I can barely comprehend now, much less as a little girl who climbed up to the top dresser drawer to make sure my test scores were good enough to make her love me.

***

SUSAN CAMERON GORMLEY.

SARAH CAMERON GORMLEY.

We are similar but not the same.

People tell me I walk like her. And that I remind them of her when I laugh, the way I throw my head back. Every once in a while, when I look in a mirror, I see Mom's blue eyes looking back at me, and I like what I see.

I am hers.

But I am not her.

PULLING ONE END OF THE RIBBON

On one of our last big family vacations in 2014—two years after I started meeting with David, two years before Dad died, and three years before I moved home—Mom and I were sitting alone in chaise lounges on a wide front porch of one of the "South Carolina Row Cottages" at a resort called the Greenbrier on a warm July afternoon. The Greenbrier was an important symbol in the family, as Mom's father started taking her and her brothers and their families there once the oil company started prospering. It was Grandpa's way of saying, *We've made it; we've earned the right to be here*, and the trips over the years served as reminders not to take our family wealth for granted. Even before people started talking about "entitlement," we knew there was nothing more disgusting.

Mom knew about my therapy by this point, that I was working through some hard things she didn't fully understand and that we weren't going to talk about, at least not directly. We talked every day, me calling between meetings or on the walk to or from the office, but I didn't share with her what David and I talked about, specifically because our work was starting to circle more closely to my relationship with her.

I don't know where everyone else was. I remember the stillness on the porch, the sound of summer across the large lawn between our house and the main hotel. I felt a calm wave of knowing between us. The ability to be quiet in the same place. I felt her looking at me, observing me from where she sat.

I didn't break the quiet as I typically might. I wanted her to see me.

Several minutes passed. Then Mom got up, walked over, and quietly kissed me on the forehead.

"I'm sorry you are hurting, honey."

"I know," I replied. At the time, I appreciated her gesture, an acknowledgment of the work I was doing in an effort to improve things in my life, for my life.

Now when I think about this scene, I recognize it as something more, as a moment of real maternal love and caring, possibly courage. She was acknowledging—and therefore admitting to herself—that her daughter was in pain, the daughter she created and lived within, and sometimes through.

I think by acknowledging my suffering and bringing it to the surface, Mom started to set me free. In this quiet moment of truth telling, I felt as if she was seeing the real me and, although I didn't need it, giving me permission to keep healing.

ABOUT CAMILLUS

It's hard to write about love because I fear I'll sound like the biggest fucking cliché surrounded by perfectly strewn rose petals. I'm afraid that's what it sounds like when I try to describe how I feel about loving him and what loving and being loved have opened up in me. On the one hand, I finally get what all of the fucking fuss is about: no wonder the best books, movies, songs, and paintings of all time usually have to do with *love*. Big love, capital-*L* love. I had no idea that the thing I wanted to save me was actually better than what I ever imagined, even though somebody else's love wasn't doing the saving. And so you ask, what did you imagine it to be? And that's the thing about spending almost your entire life in a blender of self-loathing—you can't imagine feeling good at all, ever. And then when I got my head and heart kind of right after years of therapy and even though my life seemed like a mess, right then this big love came in, seemingly out of nowhere.

Imagine that—imagine not being able to feel good about yourself and then, whammo, a massive Mack truck of healthy love comes barreling into you. I was finally ready, because I did the work. That part I get. Now, finally. I get it. No therapy, no Camillus.

I didn't know real intimacy. Sex, I did the sex part. Nailed that shit. I had lots of practice with men who didn't care what my middle name was and would never know that I struggle putting lids on things.

Camillus knows that. Camillus knocked over a Sarah-closed bottle of olive oil and claims that he smiled when he saw the small, shimmery pool forming on his pantry shelf. Is that intimacy? Damn straight.

I didn't know that somebody's wrists—*wrists*—could turn me on. He has two of them. Carpal-tunneled, ex-football-player wrists. I like to touch him. I absorb him through my hands the way I absorbed the farm through my feet as a little kid running barefoot. Don't get me started on the kissing. Even a cheek, my lips on his skin. I didn't know how love changes the physical—didn't know that comfort, lust, hunger, and electricity all live in attraction.

What I also didn't know was that none of that goodness was going to be available to me until I sorted out my own shit. Does my story work without Camillus? Probably not. Definitely not for Hallmark. If you asked me what the payoff has been for all of the work, the ten years of therapy, I wouldn't say the art gallery. I wouldn't even say finally understanding my relationship with Mom or learning to like myself. Even though all of those things have resulted from *doing the work*, love is the payoff. The best gold star of all.

And watching Camillus walk into the room and waiting to hear him say my name and feel his hands on me . . . that is what I'm here for. All of it.

VENN DIAGRAMS

"You have to do the work."

That's what people say about therapy. *You have to do the work.* What they don't add is *if you want your life to change*, but I guess that part is implied. What you don't know is what will change or how and in what order, and if you knew how long it took, you might not go at all.

I took notes on my phone when David and I talked because some of the concepts were complicated and I couldn't always remember them from session to session. I liked to go back and remind myself of important points, especially when the running loop of self-loathing started up again, or I found myself feeling like there wasn't much progress, or that progress wasn't happening fast enough. I wanted answers and solutions. I wanted to be able to check the box and get the gold star.

Nope.

We often revisited ideas from a book called *The Drama of the Gifted Child* by Alice Miller, which explores the premise that some children can be so attuned to their parents' expectations that they do whatever it takes to fulfill them. By becoming the "perfect" child, the gifted child loses, or never finds, her true self. David didn't even mention the book until almost a full year and a half after I started meeting with him, but when he did I started to feel some relief. Here was a way of understanding my dynamic with my parents that made sense. I saw how my obsession with being what I thought my parents and society wanted me to be prevented me from becoming the person I was meant to be.

I hate how mumbo jumbo "true self" and "authentic self" sound because there are so many books, talks, and aphorisms screaming at us all of the time to be these things.

"Live authentically!"

"Life is short! Be your true self!"

"The universe will open up to you when you show up as your authentic self."

That looks great on a cross-stitched pillow, but how the fuck are you supposed to get there?

I wasn't capable of understanding *any* of this until I started working with David, and I still had to take notes and study them, and still do. The notes include something he explained to me repeatedly in person when I was in New York and on the phone in sessions in San Francisco and Ohio: three things make any of us who we truly are, a Venn diagram with three overlapping circles.

"One circle is heredity—what comes from genetic makeup," David explained. "One circle is our environment—what we experience and live through. And the third circle is what we bring into the world entirely on our own, our individual star."

Of course, that third circle was the one I struggled to understand because there was no formula, science, or order to explain it. So he kept trying.

"The third circle is the good stuff, the thing that makes you distinctly you. For each person, the relative size and impact of each of the three circles differ and can change over time, but that third circle is always what makes you uniquely Sarah."

When I tried to understand what happened to me, why I felt the way I felt, and how I was lucky enough to be able to do the necessary work to change, he often referred back to the Venn diagram, pointing out that my emotional strength came from my individual star circle.

In therapy, we tried to get rid of obstacles so that my real self had a chance to shine through in the second half of my life. I imagine this like a deep-sea diver finally coming to the surface so you see her face for the first time in the sun. The crazy part is that I'm both the diver and the girl on the dock watching the new version of myself emerge.

So in my midforties, I started to see and feel parts of me I really liked. Shocking, but true. Here goes, get ready. Drumroll, please, for the inaugural written-down list of things I like about myself (Don't laugh, it's a brutal exercise. Try it sometime!): my sense of humor, my kindness, my natural empathy for others, my intelligence (gold stars, gold stars!), and my huge capacity for love that had been sitting in reserve, dormant like a sleeping bear waiting to be awakened at the end of winter. This is who I was supposed to be all along—*this girl*, the one who knows what matters and what doesn't matter, and the one who is capable of loving and being loved. Yes, there . . . I said it, I finally discovered that girl and am becoming her still, every day.

If this was fiction, our heroine would have an aha moment when everything suddenly made sense. There'd be a lightning strike perhaps or a storm cloud passing to reveal a rainbow before the credits roll, and *that's* how you'd know she figured things out, that her life was better, that she was healing. That's not how it goes in real life. The healing is messy and slow and complicated and not all that obvious most of the time. The work is not a straight path, but the work . . . works.

At least it did for me. And David and I kept dipping back into the hard stuff like that duck swimming around a pond in circles and not at all like somebody hiking the Appalachian Trail.

FOOD AND FRIENDS

"Amy McLoughlin wants to visit and bring you some potato soup," I told Mom.

I was lying in bed next to her, as she rested, not really sleeping. "I need to shut my eyes for a few minutes," she said. Her days were spent between the chair in the front room and her bed, with the only real outings from the house to the cancer center for treatments. In terms of her eating, we just kind of made it up as we went along, trying some Ensure here, some scrambled eggs there. Every once in a while, she would crave something specific like McDonald's french fries, and I'd hit the drive-through as if on a military mission.

I knew how much Mom adored Amy, who was like a sister to me. A mile away, the McLoughlins were our closest neighbors, and our families felt woven together. Mom had been a second mom to Amy and her sisters, Patty and Theresa, since childhood. I knew she would want to see Amy, but I also knew Mom was tired of what felt like an endless string of visitors, all uncertain of whether she would recover and how many more chances they might get to talk to her.

"Soup sounds good, tell her to come down," she said.

I acted as the screener, a power position I never would have asked for but one that people honored, always reaching out to me rather than calling the house phone or texting Mom directly. There was no predictable pattern to the visits, but someone showed up daily. Amy with the soup, Kathie Balderson with pimento cheese, and Jane Cardi, who traveled from West Virginia with fresh bread from a bakery in Wheeling.

Mom was so loved, period. I knew that. But in these moments, I noticed that I didn't have to be jealous or want more of Mom for myself. I could just sit there and eat pimento cheese sandwiches and be sad that Mom was dying like a normal sad daughter. What a relief it was to eat that sandwich.

Mom would sit up and eat a few spoonfuls of the potato soup, maybe a bite of the bread with butter. We kept trying to nourish her even as we sought nourishment from her for ourselves: more insights, perspectives, and life lessons. Mom let her friends love her. Even though she didn't feel well, she tried to let them have their moments with her. Mom had a short attention span for small talk even when she was healthy, so I recognized this generosity and that many of the visits were not for her sake but for theirs.

If she was asleep or didn't feel like talking, I would sit with her visitors out in the front room and try my best to answer their questions about her treatment. Nobody specifically asked about a prognosis; it was just understood that things weren't going well but that we were *trying*.

We spent several weeks in the active illusion of trying.

THE END OF A YEAR

Christmas and New Year's passed in a slow-motion blur of family traditions and our collective denial that they would be Mom's last.

We still set up the tree in its usual spot in the window seat in the kitchen—a blue spruce because she liked the short needles and how the branches stayed firm. I added hammered-brass stars I knew Mom would love that came from some fancy store called March in San Francisco. We draped white lights and red wooden beads around the branches, keeping the decoration as simple as possible, but pretty. We placed crimson, white, and pink amaryllises in the front window, the ones Mom ordered from White Flower Farm every year and timed just right so their massive blooms would be open for Christmas. The smell of her favorite Ralph Lauren holiday candles wafted throughout the first floor. The house looked and smelled like every other Christmas at the farm, even though we knew this year was different.

Did we do the tenderloin for Christmas Eve? Exchange gifts, even? I can't recall, but what I do know is that I made some type of egg casserole on Christmas morning.

"Oh, that smells so good," she said. "You're becoming a better cook."

Mom didn't eat anything, so who knows if she really liked it, but I loved the compliment anyway. She knew I'd mostly eaten out my entire adult life except for Sunday night frozen pizzas, so her comment stayed with me. When you're in that weird half-life with a dying parent, seemingly offhand comments take on more meaning.

She knew about Camillus and me and said she was happy that we were getting to know each other. She said she liked seeing me smile at the mere mention of his name and that she had not seen me light up that way with anybody else.

Mom was out of bed and talking with my high school friend Ali and me when Camillus came to pick us up to go to a party on New Year's Eve. Mom's eyes twinkled when he walked in, and she even got up out of her chair to give him a hug. Even then, I knew that her knowing him—and that Dad had known him too—mattered, that whatever was going on between us was something to treat with care.

Mom smiled at us as we got up to leave. I told her I'd be back to check in on her in a few hours, that we were just headed up to Brad's barn a mile away, so she should call or text if she needed anything.

"Camillus, you take care of these girls tonight," she said.

Taking care of somebody. Your mother. Your boyfriend. Yourself. How little we know about how much care we need for ourselves even as we give it to another person.

THE BEGINNING OF A NEW ONE

Two weeks later and six weeks into her chemo and the awful shots, we met with Dr. Wegner again so he could update us on her blood work and whether Mom's counts—things like white blood cells and tumor markers—were improving.

"I'm sorry," he said. "I know this is hard to hear, but the treatment is not working, and your numbers are not improving. The numbers are getting worse, and I can see that you're also getting weaker, so I know your quality of life is getting worse too."

I watched Mom as she listened, wondering how she would react.

She nodded at him and then looked at me.

I asked the next question. I wanted to be strong for her and wondered how this nice man and the nurse in the room with us did this every day. Yes, there had to be good cases, but how can you do this for your job, to sit there and tell people they are dying? Suddenly those big jobs marketing software, blockbuster movies, or even stylish-but-affordable pastel butter dishes for Martha Stewart seemed better than this one.

"Is there anything else we can do?" I asked.

He looked at Mom. There was something elegant about how he respected her, acknowledging that she was the patient, not me.

"Yes, there is one more option for you: super aggressive chemo," he said. "It could have bad side effects, but we could try it as the last option. We would need to start in two weeks."

Mom didn't hesitate—didn't even blink or look down at her brown Merrill slip-on shoes held up by those awkward metal plates of the wheelchair.

"If I was your mom or wife, what would you tell her to do?" she asked.

My insides folded in on themselves when he hesitated.

"I don't know, Susan. I really don't know."

I looked at Mom, eyes pleading but firm.

"Mom, if your body can take it, I think you should at least try," I said. "If you try and it makes you feel worse, we can stop, right? But it could work. Let's just try?"

I was sure she would say no, but instead she nodded at me and then looked back at Dr. Wegner.

"Let's try," she agreed.

The nurse scheduled the next appointment for 2 p.m. on January 25, 2018.

KNOWING VERSUS *KNOWING*, AGAIN

Mom came out to the front room to watch the news the morning she was supposed to start the more aggressive treatment. She had some coffee but then went back to her bed. Because it took her a little longer than normal to get herself ready and out to the car, I gave her a heads-up from the hall that we would need to leave soon.

"Mom, we need to leave here in thirty minutes or so. Let me know if you need help with anything."

I didn't hear anything back and thought she might be asleep, so I walked into the bedroom. She was awake and had the blankets pulled up high, under her chin.

"We need to leave in like twenty-five minutes, okay?"

The television was on WHIZ, the local news station that always seemed to have the most earnest, fresh-out-of-college journalism majors who were downright terrible newscasters. Mom and I liked to critique their outfits, the Bugs Bunny tie choice, in particular.

She was watching, or pretending to watch, and then dropped her arms down on the comforter before she spoke.

"I'm not going," she said from beneath the blankets.

I wasn't sure I'd heard her properly, but my heart started racing.

"Your appointment is at two," I said. "Do you not feel like you have the energy to go? Do you want me to see if we can go tomorrow?"

I stood next to her and squeezed her hand as she shook her head. My hand was a younger, healthier version of her hand, but still all veins and skinny fingers.

I didn't want to accept what I already knew. She squeezed back.

"I'm not going, Sarah," she said. "There's no reason to go through any more of that shit. I'm dying, and it's okay."

I leaned over and kissed her cheek, my heart pounding louder and heat rising up into my face.

"Are you sure?" I asked. I paused. "If you've decided, then I am not going to try to convince you otherwise, but you've got to be sure."

"I'm sure."

I had to get out of the room before I lost it, still not wanting her to see me cry, so I went to the kitchen. I tried to call Joe, then texted him, hoping he was somewhere nearby on the farm. When he called back, I urged him to come to the house as soon as he could. Even though I felt Mom was certain, I wasn't sure my accepting her decision so quickly was the right thing to do. I needed Joe to agree, and I thought about calling Jane, but I knew she might fall apart and I didn't want to disturb her at work.

Joe found us in the bedroom, me sitting in the chair I used to climb up as a little girl and Mom in bed. He sat in the window seat, closer to Mom. His eyes were red, but I could tell he was trying to be strong.

"What's going on in here? You being a little stubborn today?" he asked.

Her blue eyes sparkled. Joe and Mom had a magic of their own, a special support system for each other that didn't fit any mold. They had a penchant for pissing people off, driving trucks too fast, cussing even more, and, yes, dipping Copenhagen.

"Oh honey, I'm not being stubborn," she said. "I'm just finished pretending I'm going to get better. I'm dying, and I know it. I don't like it, and I sure as hell wish I wasn't, but it's okay. It's really okay."

Joe's legs were crossed. He took off his baseball cap, rubbed the back of his neck, and looked at me and then at the ceiling, fighting back tears.

"Sounds to me like you've decided. We're not going to push you," he said. "Shit, if we've learned anything, we know if your mind's made up, that's that."

The three of us sat there for what felt like twenty minutes but probably wasn't even one. What are you supposed to say in the moments after your mom tells you she's accepted that she's going to die? When you feel like this can't be real life, or at least not *your* life? The room was calm, and we were still us, sitting there in the most profound yet normal moment of our lives.

I couldn't take the silence.

"I'm not sure there are rules about what to say here, but what are you thinking right now?" I asked Mom.

Joe helped me out by bringing some levity into the room.

"Tell us something important at least? We know what's coming is going to suck, so you better share your wisdom with us while we have you," Joe said.

Mom smiled at us.

"I don't think I have anything too profound to share," she said. "I know that I'm not afraid. And I know I've had a sweet life. I'm not sure too many people are lucky enough to say that at the end . . . but I've had a sweet, sweet life."

I had one question for her and sincerely wanted to know her answer. It felt too soon to ask because we still had some time until the end, but still, there we were, aware of what was going to happen. I didn't want to diminish the moment with small talk about whether she needed more water or what she might like for dinner, so I asked her.

"What's one thing you've learned, your most important life lesson? Go ahead and tell us now so we don't forget," I asked.

She paused and looked at us with intent, holding eye contact first with Joe and then with me.

Had she thought about this already? Maybe? Was she going to say something about us, and how we were what mattered most? If we were in a movie, she would say something deep, but in real life, Mom wouldn't be long-winded or preachy. I had no idea what she would say, but when she said it, it felt perfectly Susan Gormley.

"Be nice," she said. "That's really it, the answer to just about everything in life. Just be fucking nice."

PHONE CALLS

I called Jane and told her about Mom's decision. She was much calmer than I expected, and I wondered if maybe I should have called her sooner. I apologized, and she told me that it was okay, she understood, and would come to the house after work to sit with Mom. Jane and Mom also had a rhythm, with regular phone calls, updates, and reports on local gossip. I saw more clearly how much Jane was her rock from day to day and had been for years, the consistent force Mom counted on.

I called the cancer center and told them Mom wouldn't be at the appointment, that there would be no more appointments.

I called the palliative care doctor, who explained a bit about home hospice and what meds and materials they would supply. I asked her how long we had, if there was some range we should be considering. I asked her what we could expect in terms of timing. Predicting death—what a fucking thing to be good at. She told me we should have some time, between two weeks and three months. I wondered if she was compensated based on accuracy or if like meteorologists, hers was a profession where you could be wrong half the time and keep your job. I felt slightly ashamed of this thought and quickly forgave myself because Mom was dying.

I called the home health agency and told them we would need somebody at the house around the clock, not just at night, which is what we had been doing so far. We wanted Sonia, Mom's favorite, during the days and Michelle for the nights. Michelle smelled like an ashtray from ten feet away, but she was strong as an ox and incredibly kind. We would pay whatever we needed to pay to make sure we had the two of them for Mom.

I called Camillus. I wanted to hear his voice most of all.

MOONLIGHT CLARITY

Later that night, after Mom was asleep, I went for a walk.

The moon illuminated the snow in the fields, the ice forming on the pond, and even my breath in the winter air as I walked down the long driveway toward the church across Clay Pike.

I no longer felt sad, at least not the kind of sadness that brought the tears in the bedroom earlier in the day. I felt present, weighted in my body. Calm somehow. I sat on the concrete step at the front door of the church and looked back at the house, taking in the beauty and majesty of the old black farmhouse on the hill as if I were looking at it for the first time.

It was Mom and Dad's only home, and now she was lying in their bed, waiting to die.

My phone buzzed.

It was a text from Diane Benincasa, who must have heard that Mom was stopping treatment. She had known Mom since she was a little girl and was one of her favorites. There's a classic story about Diane spending the weekend at the farm when she was eleven or so. When her mom called to see how things were going, Di proudly exclaimed, "It must be going okay because Susan only called me an asshole twice!"

I didn't especially feel like talking to anyone but knew she would be hurting, too, so I called her. She told me how sorry she was, asked how I was doing, and then delivered one of those well-intentioned comments people say that can land horribly: "This must be so awful, but I think she's just ready to be reunited with The Judge."

I contemplated whether to just let it go, but I couldn't. I didn't want her death to be hijacked by people trying to make themselves feel better by applying their desired order of things—the idea of Mom and Dad being together again. I knew I was being petty. But my mom was dying, so I figured I had the right to be just a little bit petty. She was ready to die because she accepted her fate and wanted to die at home, with a modicum of dignity and not in a god-awful hospice facility.

"You know, Di," I said. "I can see why you might say that, but that's not what's happening. Mom loves life. She's not ready to die because she wants to be with Dad. She's ready to die because she has cancer all over her body."

Di and I had known each other and loved each other long enough that she knew not to argue with me. And I knew that she and others would continue to tell themselves the reunion-with-Dad story to make their loss easier to bear. I wanted to be kind and understanding, to let them do whatever they needed for their own pain. But I was also pissed off and wanted them to get their own therapists and do their own work and learn to accept that life is messy and hard, that people fucking die, and not try to tie up Mom's death with a red happily-ever-after bow. Fuck that. No more myths about Mom. I could tell Di thought I was being combative, and she probably excused my gruffness given the situation. She told me she loved me and that she would be in touch.

As I looked at the house, sounds of childhood surrounded me and memories started to fill up my veins. Truck tires on a gravel road. Cows bellowing for their babies. Summer whip-poor-wills. Somebody mowing hay in the field. Children's voices. Laughter. Kicking cinders from the bridge and awaiting the splash when they hit the water of Salt Creek, where Mom wanted her ashes to be spread from one of the blue Maxwell House coffee cans Dad used to collect his loose change in. Jane, Joe, and I playing with the hose in the front yard, then sitting at the kitchen table eating ice cream, our spoons scraping the bottom of the floral porcelain bowls. These scenes flowed over and into each other, moving throughout my body like individual movies playing out simultaneously, adding up inside me.

Mom was there, too, walking from one room of the house into another, looking for us.

AND SOMEHOW, LOVE

I know there was a time when Camillus was not part of my life.

And I know there was a time when Camillus became part of my life.

But I cannot recall any transition period or anything that felt like dating, at least not how I'd experienced dating before. I wasn't filled with uncertainty, confusion, or frustration about what he said or didn't say, when he called or didn't call, and I didn't even speculate about whether we had a potential future.

I didn't need to sit with my friends over too many glasses of wine and dissect what was going on with Camillus.

We just worked.

He had his kids every other week. During the weeks they weren't staying with him, I would drive over some nights so we could go out or make dinner together. We perfected cooking New York strip steaks in his grandmother's cast-iron skillet. He teased me about putting ice in my wine. We talked about everything and nothing until I would start falling asleep, always before him. I liked feeling his body next to me, waking up some mornings to find him watching me, knowing he was waiting for me to open my eyes.

We both knew that he was an escape for me and that I might be one for him, but we didn't talk about that or what would happen next or what this thing was between us. We didn't have to name anything.

We were just together. And just as easily and naturally as reaching over to unlock the passenger door, Camillus and I started to love each other.

HIGHWAY MUSIC

I'm on Route 161 driving home to the farm, away from Camillus and back to Mom, as she's lying at home dying from cancer, when a song from the country band LANCO comes on, the one with the lyrics that seemed as if they were written just for us.

"Friday night lights decide your fate," they sang. Camillus, the high school football star. Camillus Musselman. I'm not far from where he grew up, where every fall Friday night at Newark Catholic High School was his night. I couldn't believe I found him and that he had come into my life now. His wrists turn me on more than any man's whole being ever has, so I think this must be lust, not love—that maybe I want so badly to be away from my dying mother that I fantasize about his football-player wrists.

"Every time you smile, I know why I'm here." I'm embarrassed. Who falls in love when her mother is dying? What's wrong with me?

"I was a wild child between lost and found. Then you spoke my name, it was a sweet sound." I see him falling in love with me and feel it on his breath when he says my name. He says my name all of the time, likes saying my name, and calls me Sarah more than he needs to, when I know he's talking to me—of course he's talking to me because I'm the only other person in the room. When he says my name, he's saying it for him, but when I hear him saying it, I feel it healing me. Like he's recognizing me as I'm finally recognizing myself. I feel like me. But Mom is dying. Fuck. Mom is dying.

"Rescue kiss and you pulled me in. All my life baby, where you been?" I've been trying so hard to be somebody else that I don't even know where I've been. I've lived in Chicago, New York, and San Francisco. I've lived in so many places, but I've never felt at home with myself, and in myself, until now.

I feel like I'm home when he's next to me. Camillus feels like home. I wonder if he's been waiting for me, if the universe has aligned just for us somehow, but then think this is not Hallmark. This is real life. Mom is dying. Mom is dying. How can this be happening? When this song ends, when will I hear the lyrics again? How can I keep hearing this song, the one I'm in with him, because I love hearing him say my name, even when he doesn't need to?

If Camillus just keeps saying my name, I might be able to stay alive even when Mom dies.

TALKING ABOUT LOVE

I wanted to tell the truth, and I wanted David to like Camillus. Not like I wanted friends to like guys I dated, but because David knew the cleaned-up mess of me better than anyone else. We'd been working together for five years, and sometimes he felt like a friend. I wanted him to approve of something that felt so unusual—and good—to me.

I told him how kind Camillus was, how much I liked just talking with him, and how thoughtful and incredibly sensitive this big, redneck-looking, manly man could be, hoping David would come back with "He might be the one!"

David never took the bait. He kept pushing me with questions about how *I was feeling* and why *I thought I was feeling things*, so I might understand myself better. I told him what I'd been thinking, and I thought it sounded significant, profound even.

"Camillus makes me feel like a better version of myself," I said.

I should have anticipated the reminder from David about something we had been talking about for years, but I had slipped into my romance novel mode for a minute.

"Well, that sounds wonderful, but of course, nobody can make you feel something about yourself, Sarah," he pointed out. "This topic usually comes up when people blame others for making them 'feel bad' about themselves, but I think it's worth pointing out in this context too."

I knew how much I'd sought external validation my entire life, and appreciated the risk of handing off this power to other people, but I thought when the result was positive, it might make more sense. Camillus *did* make me feel good about myself, so why was David nitpicking? I was frustrated, especially because I felt like I was so close to getting the gold star for love and just wanted David to be happy for me.

"I don't know, but he *does* make me feel better about myself!"

I could almost hear his slow pause.

"Let's go slowly," he said.

He always said this when we were revisiting a topic or going into something he knew I struggled with, and in this case the challenge was both me acknowledging and maybe taking some credit for the progress I'd made in our work together. I probably mouthed the words "Let's go slowly" and rolled my eyes to myself.

"Try telling me how you feel about yourself when you're with Camillus," he said. "Not how he 'makes' you feel, but how you feel."

I paused for a long time. I could feel the heat rising up into my face and the tears welling up.

"I don't know," I said. "I feel like me, but a better version of me. Comfortable. I don't hesitate or overthink what I'm going to say. I don't do that thing where I'm watching and judging myself through the lens of the imaginary cameraman across the room. I almost feel like I'm kind of cool, like somebody I might want to hang out with. Does that make sense?"

David laughed even though I wasn't trying to be funny.

"Yes, that makes sense, and I'm guessing there might be lots of people who would like to hang out with you," he said. "What else can you tell me about when you're with him? Say more."

There it was: the say-more directive I'd come to expect from him. "This is super embarrassing, but I feel like a girl somehow," I said. "I feel feminine and, yes, even pretty. There, I said it, okay? I feel pretty when I'm with Camillus."

"Wow," he said. "You're starting to sound a lot like a person who likes herself."

Cue the tears.

When you've spent your whole life disliking yourself and your therapist points out that maybe you finally *do* like yourself, that you've crossed over into that foreign, far-off land reserved only for fairy tales and mythical creatures, it's a pretty big deal.

The shift didn't happen at that exact moment, of course, but hearing something spoken aloud is powerful and brought the reality of my change to the surface in a new way. The shift had been happening for years, ever since our first session. David slowly guided me toward a new understanding of myself that was far healthier, but it took time.

Change is not a lightning bolt.

Change is not a straight hike.

Change doesn't happen in order.

Change is laps around the same pond, finding nourishment in new ways.

Change is the daily reminder that I deserve to feel good about myself.

I have no idea why it's so much easier to hate ourselves than to love ourselves, and feeling good about myself still makes me cringe sometimes, like a sweater that's a little too tight regardless of how flattering. *Am I going to wear this out in public? What if somebody sees me in this thing?*

And even though he would never come out and say so, I swear David was secretly hoping for Camillus and me to win the Big Love Cook-Off.

WRITING ABOUT ALL OF IT

You've made it this far into the book you are holding in your hands, so maybe by now I should feel comfortable calling myself a writer. I wanted to tell you this story about me, about Mom, about love and grief and hope, and I wanted to make sense of things by writing them all down.

I believe I wanted to write before I knew how to write.

I know this because there's a photo of me as a toddler, sitting in front of Grandma Gormley's typewriter.

Gray and bulky and heavy, the typewriter had keys that jumped up to imprint the paper and sometimes got stuck. I remember prying them back with my small fingers to start over. I loved the sound of the space bar and each metal key striking the paper, leaving behind letters that I knew meant something to grown-ups. When the photo was taken, I had a bad cold, and you can see the snot filling in the space between my nose and upper lip. My short white-blond hair looks damp and a little sweaty, my cheeks red with a slight fever.

Grandma took the photo because she wanted to capture how I looked when I informed her with great certainty that I was going to write a letter to Mom and Dad.

I didn't feel well, and I wanted them to come get me.

I wanted to write because I wanted to go home.

I thought writing might save me.

***

I don't want to write what comes next.

I've been thinking about this part of the book since I wrote the first sentence of the prologue, before I first admitted how much and for how long I hated myself, before I showed you the farm, before I introduced my college friends, and before I struck the keys to spell *C-a-m-i-l-l-u-s* for the first time.

This is when life changes.

This is when Mom dies.

I've been not writing this part for weeks, sitting in reluctance, drafting scenes in my head, but not putting anything on the page, unwilling to create potential permanence with each letter of this part of my story.

I don't want to write this part because I'm afraid.

I'm afraid I'm going to forget something she said. I'm afraid I'm going to leave out an important detail about the way the kitchen smelled when I reheated stale coffee rather than making a fresh pot. Or the way her skin felt, so smooth and loose, like something you could unwrap, the physical gift of her life.

I'm afraid that when I stop writing this part, she really will be gone.

I'm afraid I won't be able to get her back.

I don't want to write the next part because I'm afraid to lose Mom.

And I know that writing won't save her.

A WEEK BEFORE SHE DIES

We were headed into the fourth week since the palliative care doctor told us we would have two weeks to three months before she died. If the doctor's range was accurate, would we have two more months, two more weeks, or two more days? The calendar makes no sense when you're in this death limbo, except that with each passing day, you're acutely aware that you're one day closer to the last.

Planning her funeral felt less absurd now—more practical than anything.

Although I still didn't particularly want to write the obituary with her, I asked her to approve one line of what would be an extremely straightforward obituary:

In August 1963, Susan married Joseph A. Gormley, with whom she enjoyed fifty-three years of lively and loving partnership marked by much humor and laughter.

She smiled and gave me a thumbs-up when I read it to her. As she got increasingly tired and weak, she started using thumbs-up and thumbs-down in response to questions.

"The thumbs-down thing is pretty dramatic, don't you think?"

"Well, I'm dying, so maybe I'm permitted to be dramatic, don't you think?"

She was right, so we continued the planning.

"Maxwell House coffee can for your ashes, no casket?"

Thumbs-up.

"Service at Grace United Methodist, with Vince Cardi doing the eulogy?"

Thumbs-up.

"Food and drinks for family and friends at Bryan Place afterward?"

Sarcasm-laced thumbs-down.

When we discussed it earlier, she told us she did not want people to gather for food and drinks afterward, but Jane convinced her that people would want to visit and tell their stories about how *wonderful* and *amazing* she was, and Mom acquiesced.

She then suggested that everything should be by invitation only. We asked her why, and her answer was just about the most Susan Gormley thing I'd ever heard.

"I don't want anyone I don't like to be there."

SIX DAYS BEFORE SHE DIES

Whether it was this day or a few days before I cannot recall; I just know there was a lot of snow. So much snow that Michelle, the night nurse, wasn't sure she could make it up the driveway because she had a spare tire on what she called her "shitty little car." Joe instructed her to go to City Tire and that he would pay for them to replace the spare. When she got there, they told her Joe had called and said, rather than just the one, he wanted to buy her four new tires. Michelle was in tears when she arrived that night, saying that nobody had ever done something so nice for her, which made me wonder how she had grown up to do a job that required a level of kindness and generosity I wouldn't have been able to imagine until I experienced it myself. I knew how generous Joe was, that we had always been taught to be growing up, but I also knew that what we wanted most was for Mom's care not to be interrupted. If Michelle needed to be airlifted in via helicopter every night, he might have paid for that too.

We wanted Mom to be as okay as she could be, and these women, Michelle and Sonia, saved us. They made the days and nights bearable for Mom, and therefore, for us.

Saint Sonia. She always just knew—what to say, what to do, how to handle Mom when she needed to be handled, and how to handle us. Some mornings, Mom would wake up before she arrived and would ask me, "Where is she? When is Sonia getting here?" Sonia wore navy scrubs and had long, beautiful red hair that she kept pulled back or up in a bun. She wasn't tall and was a little bit stout, with a wonderful laugh you could hear from the kitchen when she was in the bedroom with Mom.

I had no idea you could come to trust and love somebody so quickly in such a singular, pure way until I met Sonia. We didn't know much about her (although she did tell us about her daughter and her dogs), but we depended on her. The relief her presence brought to the farm was palpable, as if the entire house exhaled when Sonia walked in. We knew that no matter what happened on any particular day, Sonia would make it okay somehow.

FIVE DAYS BEFORE SHE DIES

Sonia told me Mom's oxygen level was low and that it was time for a catheter. She was too weak to get to the bathroom and back and wasn't always able to tell Sonia in time to help get her there. The hospice service from the hospital came out to count the pills and deliver supplies, and when I got back from the grocery store, Mom was hooked up to the oxygen and had the catheter in place. One day closer to the last.

I got into bed with her to take a little nap, intending to see Camillus that night. Mom and I had talked about whether she wanted me to stay at the farm every night. For the last few weeks she'd insisted I continue to drive over and stay with him. She told me she thought it was important that we had time to be alone together, that couples needed that time.

Except not that night.

"Sarah, I think you better stay here tonight," she said.

I wondered what was going on—why she suddenly needed me more.

"Of course," I said. "What did you have in mind? Do you think we should go out dancing or maybe have a *Little House on the Prairie* marathon?"

I definitely don't think we're the funniest family around, but our attempts at humor made some of the most god-awful scenes you could ever live through more palatable, and I knew Mom agreed with me.

Thumbs-down.

"No, I don't think we're going to do any of that," she said. "I think I'm going to die tonight."

I knew a little bit about how the dying thing goes, after being with Dad near the end—about the death rattle and the dark spots on the skin, the markers that death was coming soon. I also knew her vitals were still pretty good because Sonia had told us just two hours earlier, so while I didn't want to disagree with a dying woman who had just announced she was going to die *that night*, I didn't think it seemed likely.

"Um, okay, I don't mean to be rude, but I don't think you just get to decide when you're going to die," I said. "Or maybe you do? Don't you remember how long it took with Dad? Plus, you're lying here still talking to me, and if it's okay with you, I'd like to do the same thing tomorrow."

Thumbs-up.

She didn't die that night. But I knew she was ready, really ready. Just in case, I sent the texts and made the calls and informed the right people that if Mom had it her way, she was going to die.

FOUR DAYS BEFORE SHE DIES

I woke up before her the next morning.

I'd slept with her and held her hand as she fell asleep just in case, and because, well, if there was anyone who *could* will herself to die, it would be Susan Gormley. I waited for her to open her eyes and gave her the most shit-eating grin I could muster.

"Well, good morning, sunshine," I said.

"Fuck you," she replied.

"Cool it," I said. "You can't be mad at me because you're still alive. I'm not in charge here and neither are you. Chocolate or vanilla?"

I turned on the *Today* show, got her a vanilla Ensure, and went upstairs to take a shower.

I let myself cry in the shower sometimes, to let out the stress and the pain I didn't want Mom to see. On the one hand, she expected that this would be hard on us, but I hated the idea of our hurting making it worse for *her*. I figured having to die was bad enough, really, so why should she have to see her children falling apart?

I remember reaching out to hold myself up on the wall as the hot water streamed down my back and realizing that the tears weren't just about losing her. This was different. I was somehow completely aware of how lucky we were to have each other and to be doing this awful thing *this way*.

We had the financial means to get extra help. We had a great family, both our immediate family and the Cameron cousins, not to mention the friends who were so close, they were like our family. We were part of an actual community. The small town I couldn't wait to leave as a child now became a comfort that showed up as food and calls and messages and immediate responses to any request.

Watching a parent die is awful and shitty and terrible and one of the worst things that you'll ever do—twice if you have two parents—and yet, you can still feel incredibly fortunate.

The emotional stew was exhausting, and I wasn't sure how or if I could sustain it much longer. But I didn't have a choice.

I wasn't in charge of this part.

For a long time, I tried to control my life for specific outcomes, and even when my plans didn't seem to work very well, I kept trying to maintain the proper order, including how I reacted when things went poorly. I internalized and rationalized and figured out how to blame myself for both my lack of control and what I thought was my weakness when I couldn't be happy with the way things were. And now, here I was, in control of absolutely nothing, 100 percent in the thick of both major personal unknowns and our ensuing loss, and what I felt wasn't anger or blame or even sadness.

As I turned my face up toward the showerhead and let the water rinse the salty rivulets of tears from my cheeks and down my chin and my neck, I realized this strange but calming feeling was gratitude. Slowly and powerfully, without urgency or alarm, gratitude started filling in the spaces previously reserved for pain.

THREE DAYS BEFORE SHE DIES

"Guess what, Mama Sue? The girls are coming to see you tomorrow."

She hated being called Sue or Susie and anything but Susan, so I liked to wind her up from time to time with a good Mama Sue zinger.

"Oh, good. I can't wait to get my hands on them." Another Susan Gormley line that was both metaphorical and quite literal.

The girls were Nancy, Tippett, and Brooks, my DePauw girls. They wanted to see her, so they were coming to the farm. Looking back, I know they also were coming to see me.

This is what we do for each other. We go. We get on the plane. We make the long drive. We put our own lives on hold because when one of us needs the others, we show up. Without question and without complaint, we prioritize each other again and again because this kind of friendship is both life-giving and lifesaving. We've talked about how we haven't taken each other for granted, not once, since the days of drinking beer and putting crumpled dollar bills into the jukebox at a dive bar called the Nisei in Chicago.

Later that afternoon, I went into the bedroom to see if she needed anything.

She was on top of the covers in just an oversized T-shirt and her underwear, kind of lifting up her legs one at a time. With the catheter tube and the oxygen, she looked as if she was practicing some type of strange bed aerobics.

"What are you doing?" I asked.

"I don't know," she responded. "I'm just tired of sitting here."

It wasn't especially cold that day. The sun was shining, and the farm looked beautiful. I thought maybe we could go outside just for a little while.

"Do you want to bundle up and go outside? You could get some fresh air?"

I was met with a thumbs-down.

Another moment of heart-sinking awareness of what was going on, how much closer we must be. Mom was always a person who was up for going on an adventure and trying something new. She said yes more than she said no. She loved to be outside. This was another instance of knowing what I didn't want to know. There had been many of these, and I'd arrived at a point where I couldn't unknow what was happening. I didn't cry and didn't walk out of the room this time. I just said okay and accepted that she might never leave the farmhouse again.

I walked toward her bed to plant a little kiss on her forehead, and she told me she wanted to show me something. She circled her hands around the upper part of her right thigh, fingers easily touching, if not overlapping.

"Look how skinny I am."

I gave her my most are-you-fucking-kidding-me look, and inside I felt my sinking heart swell with appreciation. I knew her comment wasn't truly her exulting in her thinness—although I suspected there was a hint of that somehow, given she had always been a professional dieter. It was about the absurdity of this situation. She said what she said *for me*, to make me laugh to save me with our special formula of love wrapped in humor, as we did again and again for each other.

"Oh yes, you're definitely super skinny," I joked back. "Cancer is a fantastic diet, isn't it?"

Thumbs-up.

TWO DAYS BEFORE SHE DIES

Nobody knew Mom was going to die two days later.

"Girls, get in here so I can get my hands on you," Mom said, summoning them into her bed. She managed one of her signature Susan Gormley lines even with the oxygen tube that never stayed in place. She constantly fidgeted with it and kept asking the nurse if she could take the damn thing out, as if the oxygen tube was the problem and not the cancer.

Mom called us all "girls," and although we were women given our fortysomething calendar years, we still felt like the girls who met at DePauw University, when our greatest responsibility was figuring out which dive bar to go to on Thursday night.

The February morning light poured into the room from over the hillside dotted with black cows, whose breath made small clouds in the winter air. I sat in the window seat closest to Mom's side of the bed and watched the girls climb up on her left side. They looked as if they were playing follow-the-leader, one behind the next, without a second of apprehension.

"Oh, look at you, my faves came to see me." Mom's usual curse-laden big voice was now like faint bursts of whisper between strained breaths.

Brooks couldn't give Mom one of the squeeze-the-air-out-of-you hugs she's been known for since we lived on the third floor of Mason Hall our freshman year, when she somehow landed in the Indiana cornfields from Tampa, Florida, all Laura Ashley one-piece jumpers and brown curls. Her Southern manners barely concealed a bawdy sense of humor and penchant for Bud Light back then, and now here she was, touching Mom's shoulder as she kissed her on the cheek. "Hi, honey," Brooks said. Mom called everyone she loved "honey," and as an unspoken honorific, we all called her the same thing in return.

Mom got to know these girls in a timeline that mirrored my own. Once I moved away from the farm, and even after college, I spoke to her every day. That was our routine. I'd give her all of the news from our first apartments in Chicago to various boyfriends and bad dates. Mom knew who hated her job, who got a bad haircut, and which one was told she could only eat bagels and bananas if she wanted to stop shitting so much. Mom knew these things because I told her, and over time, the girls became hers too.

I looked at Tippett next to Brooks on the bed. Her father died our sophomore year, and I wondered how being here felt for her. I remembered when she came to visit the farm over Labor Day weekend when we were in our late thirties. We sat down in the garden, where Mom was holding court, a glass of Chardonnay in hand.

"Tell us what it was like growing up with a father who was a professor." Mom had never met Mr. Tippett, but rather than making small talk about this recipe or that child's activity, she created a space to talk about something that mattered. What I remember most was Tippett's eyes lighting up in appreciation for Mom's asking, and then, for her listening.

In the bedroom, Mom was observing her. "Tippett, you are so beautiful. And all of you girls are. Have you always been this beautiful, or have I forgotten?" Of course, Mom had never worn a stitch of makeup and at least claimed that looks didn't matter, but I wondered if being so close to their youth and vibrancy felt like a spotlight on her frailty.

Still a tomboy at heart, Nancy climbed up onto the bed wearing her Saucony sneakers that looked just like the pair she was wearing the night I introduced her to her future husband, Don, a family friend. Mom was like his second mom, which extended a thick layer of loyalty and love to Nancy. Nancy patted Mom's leg and gave her a big, toothy smile with her eyebrows raised up. "Susan, you know we like to be told we're beautiful, but we're not here to talk about us. We just want to sit here with our best gal. Sarah has been keeping us updated, and we think this whole situation sucks."

I swallowed hard when she called me "Sarah," the first time I'd heard Nancy call me anything other than "Gorms" since freshman year. I wondered if Mom noticed. Rather than teasing about the formality, she stayed quiet and nodded with what looked like a reluctant mix of agreement and acquiescence. Mom and I had talked about how much time she might have, but watching her admit to somebody else what was happening took my breath away. The girls were now witnesses, and my heart swelled in my body.

I thought about us dancing in front of the funky soul band playing "Shout" at Don and Nancy's wedding. Mom bounded onto the floor, arms flying in the air and her white hair wet with sweat from a dance style that was more exuberance than skill. In the video from that night, you can see us watching Mom from our table at the edge of the parquet dance floor, laughing at first, then realizing it might look like we are laughing at her. Then one by one we jumped in right next to her, flailing our own arms in the highest form of flattery.

Even though I'd often felt jealous when Mom doted on other people, with the girls it was different—more like the love multiplied between us. I loved seeing her love them even knowing it might be the last time.

Mom's eyes fluttered between open and closed, and I moved to sit next to her right side. I took her right hand in mine and noticed how much they looked alike, even though hers seemed smaller, childlike. I could feel her trying to tell me something. The girls were still there, the three of them on the other side of her body, like a small chorus watching Mom and me.

She reached out her other hand and gently touched my nose with her index finger. She'd never touched me this way before. At first, I thought she was saying *I see you* or *I know you*. But she was trying to make a point.

She then took the same finger and touched her own nose. In the faintest but clearest voice, she said one word.

"Lucky."

Lucky. I let the word wash over me. I wanted Mom to know I'd heard her, and I repeated it back.

"Lucky."

When I said it, I felt as if I was signing a contract between us.

The knowledge of what was happening, and how close we were getting to the end, could have filled this moment with profound sadness. But the word felt like an exhale, an observation that was expansive, not final. Before I could make sense of what she meant, she let go of my hand and her head sank back farther into the pillow.

"I need to shut my eyes."

The girls and I knew it was time to leave, so we walked out to the kitchen without saying goodbye, the way you tiptoe out of a room when a baby falls asleep.

We stood there, quiet, with the shared knowledge that something profound had just happened. We were little girls who didn't know what to do next and women who knew exactly what to do next. But we were still us, and the poignancy was light. Nancy broke the silence.

"Jesus, Gorms, you could have warned us. That was rough. Good grief."

I wouldn't have it any other way.

Looking back, I see how Mom's one-word declaration was about the two of us being lucky to have each other, but it was also about her certainty that the girls would keep holding me up. Their presence that morning reassured her, and I now imagine a handoff taking place, as if being able to assign me to them made it easier for her to get closer to death.

***

These days and hours passed in a surreal loop where time didn't really stand still, but there seemed to be no point when one day ended and the next began. I only know what happened on what day because I looked back at the calendar and figured out the sequence of events.

Things just happened. Days unfolded.

That evening we went to Joe and Christi's house—ten minutes away if you took a buggy—for lasagna so we wouldn't be too far away from Mom.

I imagined how we must look that night from the outside, if somebody was up on the hill, looking down at the cozy scene, the white candlelight illuminating our faces as we laughed, drinking beer and wine and talking about Mom while not really talking about what was happening. I imagined we looked like we were celebrating something special, like a scene from the opening credits of a movie that made you want to be a part of the friendship and warmth, having no idea that the guests were in town to visit their friend's dying mother.

We knew Sonia would text if anything developed, and when I checked in with her, she let us know that Mom was sleeping.

I'm sure I drank too much red wine that night and maybe smoked too much pot, although during that period no amount of wine or weed seemed to make me feel bad the next day, like my body was on cruise control and kept going to sleep and waking up early the next day with no recollection of bad decisions the night before. It felt as if my mind knew not to be judgmental about anything going on with me physically, as if my emotional control center had sent a don't-fuck-with-us-right-now memo to excuse all of the excesses.

THE DAY BEFORE SHE DIES

We woke up Saturday and Mom was worse, even though *worse* feels like the wrong word. Maybe she was *declining* or *failing*, but even those words felt insufficient and so negative when what was happening was that her body was getting closer to death. Fewer breaths. Fewer minutes with her eyes open. And even though she was so frail, there seemed to be a heaviness to her form in the bed, as if death was entering and her body was getting ready.

Jane came down early that morning to see Mom and say hi to my friends, and when she came out of the bedroom, she made a face as her eyes welled up.

"She's not in very good shape, is she?" she asked.

I hated this for Jane and realized that she had a hard time sitting with Mom knowing she was dying. She was far better than Joe and me in a hospital and spent many more hours visiting with Dad throughout his various stays, but Jane was different here. Even though we were all glad she was at home, I sensed that seeing Mom was too painful for her, because she always changed the subject to mundane tasks of her day, like what she needed from the grocery store, and she usually didn't stay very long.

My sadness for my siblings during this time was powerful, held together by a unique thread of appreciation, memories of weeknights at the dinner table, and an adult understanding that grief was different for each of us.

I hated that Jane was in pain, and I didn't want her to feel guilty about leaving.

"No, she's not. I think we're getting close. Go home and do whatever you need to do. I'll call you if anything changes," I told her.

Mom wasn't able to talk much, and her breath was shallow. Sometimes her eyes fluttered between open and closed when she tried to talk to us. The girls and I went in to say hello, and I remember I took in a cup of coffee because she said she still liked the smell.

We told her about dinner the night before, that Christi's lasagna was delicious, and that we had a nice visit and talked about her *the whole time*.

***

I want to tell you the things that matter—to show you what the days looked like and how it felt to be in this strange half-life of loss and love.

I fear I'm failing you, that I'm forgetting little things that maybe don't matter but somehow do, like the fact that the ice maker stopped working, and how much Mom hated dealing with machines that stopped working and how she wouldn't have to deal with that ice maker ever again.

Looking back, I can see that as my mom was dying in the other room, I escaped into minutiae like the ice maker and allowed myself to laugh about Tippett's hot-rod rental car because I had to laugh, as the days kept coming and I had to do all of the things that made up any day, like showering and eating and sleeping.

Something happens in the days surrounding such loss that suspends the order of things, as if time is holding its own breath to permit you to forget, if even for a few minutes, the very thing that is happening. At the same time, you're keenly aware of the absurd beauty of being there, as if you're constantly observing yourself from the outside, confirming that this is happening, that this is your life.

***

That Saturday was oddly warm for February in Ohio, and the boys decided we should take advantage of the sunshine and go for a buggy ride. In hindsight, I can see that the physical activity—being outside, away from her bedroom—was a way to escape the sadness, even if only for a few hours. We had observed Mom's pragmatic approach to Dad's death, so there was no guilt about not sitting next to her for hours on end. In fact, we knew she would be pissed if we kept vigil at her bedside.

Sometimes I still look at the photos from that day.

Brooks drinking a can of Miller Lite in coveralls with a big hole in the ass where a previous wearer likely stood too close to a campfire.

Tippett sitting next to Camillus in his buggy, her eyes wide, trying to look excited even though she probably was slightly terrified as they headed down a steep hill.

Brooks riding with Joe toward the cave, his face bright with affection for her and pride about the farm, probably telling her something about the property or when he first started making the trails that laced the woods.

Brooks, Tippett, and me standing in the cave, with the not-yet-spring waterfall splashing down behind us. It's the same cave Camillus and I visited during the Cooner so many years before. The girls had heard about him, of course, and once they met him, they quickly understood this thing that had formed between us.

***

After the buggy rides, we decided to check in on Mom, to see if we might be able to make her smile, to make sure she knew we were right there.

Joe sat next to her, and I could see that this was their moment. I wasn't sure she was aware that we were in the room. She started singing to him a song I'd never heard her sing, in a sweet and soft voice, tapping his arm as she sang.

"I love you, a bushel and a peck . . ."

From where I was sitting, I could see the tears start streaming down Joe's face.

"A bushel and a peck and a hug around the neck . . ."

Joe tried to stop himself from crying by taking deep breaths.

"Don't stymie them, it's okay to cry, honey," she said.

Mom was firm, strong, and clear. She knew what she wanted to say and wanted him to understand, and I felt myself in awe of her grace.

I love you a bushel and peck . . .

A bushel and a peck and a hug around the neck . . .

We managed to get ourselves out of the room and leave Joe and Mom alone for a few more minutes. Tippett, Brooks, Camillus, and I were in the kitchen, trying to recover from what we'd just witnessed. I wondered if they felt that they shouldn't have been in the room with us, that it was too much. I didn't want them to feel uncomfortable.

Years later, Brooks told me she considered being there with us one of the greatest gifts she'd ever received.

THE DAY SHE DIES

Back in the bedroom, Sonia was trying to get Mom to swallow something, probably a pain pill, but it wasn't working. She said she would call hospice and have them bring syringes, but for now we could crush the pills into something easy for her to swallow, like pudding.

We didn't have any pudding.

Camillus and Brad were in the kitchen. Brad had been bringing donuts to the farm every Sunday morning for fifteen years. That was his routine, and Mom was still alive, so there he was with a box of Donald's Donuts, including Mom's favorite, a plain old-fashioned stick.

Just as I was telling them I needed to run to the grocery store to get some pudding, I saw a car coming up the driveway. We realized it was Susan Benincasa, Don and Diane's mom and Nancy's mother-in-law, who had a penchant for small talk. Mom adored her, but today was not the right day. Not for me.

I was in no mood to be nice to anyone—or talk to anyone or even *see* anyone—and I knew Camillus could see my mood shifting. His truck was parked directly in front of the house, and the ground was soft given the warm weather and melting snow, so he and Brad went outside to make sure Susan didn't try to drive her little Mercedes through the field.

Sonia came out to the kitchen, and I told her what was going on.

"Susan Benincasa is coming up the driveway, and I need to get the fuck out of here right now."

We looked out the window just in time to see the boys pointing, signaling to her to stay on the driveway, which she seemed to ignore, pulling directly onto the soft grass of the field, where the Mercedes immediately sank into the damp, soft ground.

Sonia and I looked at each other and laughed a little, shaking our heads in disbelief, but now Susan was walking toward the front door. She had a tiny little white fur jacket on, which I found infuriating, as somehow in my Mom-dying logic I didn't think a little white fur jacket was the thing to wear when you show up uninvited and unannounced to the farmhouse for this occasion.

The wheels were almost entirely off my wagon by this point.

Sonia could see what was happening.

"Go out the kitchen door, and I'll meet her at the front door. You won't even have to talk to her. Go!" she said.

I did what she said, and walked over to the barn as Susan went into the house, not even seeing me, as if I was crossing behind her on stage. Camillus and Brad were attaching a chain to the tractor to pull Susan's car out of the mud. I climbed into Camillus's truck, wondering how mean I just was, realizing that Susan was suffering too.

But I didn't care.

I had to go to town to buy pudding to help get morphine into my dying mother.

***

Camillus, Brad, and I drove to the grocery store, the same place where I did parking-lot therapy with David every Tuesday. I stood in an aisle looking at packages of pudding. I thought about chocolate or vanilla, recalling how Mom would make pudding the old-fashioned way on the stove when we were little, how it seemed like it took forever for it to cool down enough for us to eat. I bought a pack of vanilla and a pack of chocolate, completely aware that Mom would never live long enough to eat that much pudding.

Outside, Camillus was waiting for me.

"How are you doing?" he asked.

"Not good at all. I'm about to lose it. Just get me to the truck."

I climbed into the back seat just as it started. A sob came out that sounded like a howl from my core. Brad got out but Camillus stayed there in the truck, reaching his hand back to touch my knee but staying quiet. I let my head fall down between my knees, let the howl come out, let myself feel the pain coming through my body, the physical realization of what I knew was happening intellectually, what I had known for the week before, the month before, the three months before but didn't want to accept. My body took over. A reconciliation was taking place inside me, like my body knew I had to let the pain come out. There was nothing to figure out. I just had to feel.

Once the wave passed, I felt a sense of relief, like I could take a breath. I looked at Camillus, who was watching me. When our eyes met, I felt stronger, as if I was borrowing his strength.

***

By the time we got home, the hospice team from the hospital had delivered the syringes and Sonia had given Mom the morphine. I remember thinking the syringes seemed tiny, too small to contain enough morphine to eliminate what I imagined must be an inordinate amount of pain. We knew the cancer was all over her spine, but I now pictured it spread throughout her body, thick and heavy.

The last day was filled with different faces sitting around the kitchen table—people who wanted to help but didn't know what they could do to help; people who loved Mom and wanted to provide some comfort if they could.

I tried to be nice even though I felt like taking a nap and waking up when everything was over. Which is exactly what Mom would have wanted to do. The thought of her saying, "I need to take a nap, my bed is calling," made me smile, and I started to understand she would always be able to make me smile.

The afternoon faded into early evening.

Then the rattle started. The god-awful death rattle. The sound you can't unhear. The sound Joe and I decided should be the soundtrack for every horror movie ever made.

I was worried about Sonia, which was kind of fucked up. I certainly don't think I'm the nicest person in the world, but I kept worrying about other people, even the nurse whose assignments concluded when her patients died. She knew what was coming, but I could see how special Mom was to her—that in her own way, she loved Mom too. When she told us she expected that Mom would die that night, I could see that she had been crying.

After the small talk, the last goodbyes back in the bedroom, and the final walks back out to the kitchen on the creaking floorboards near the fireplace, the house started to empty.

Eventually, Jane and Joe left too. I told them I would call them. The decision was pragmatic because there wasn't anything more we could do but wait, and I didn't feel as if all of us had to be there. I wasn't trying to be a martyr, although on some level, I thought because I had been there with Dad when he died, I knew I wanted to be there with Mom too. I think each of us had our own struggle with how we wanted to remember her, and seeing a body after death is not easy to unsee. I was happy to take on the role if it might save Jane and Joe from seeing her that way.

I knew these things, and I felt calm and clear.

In no small way, Mom helped us prepare—she had been helping us prepare for the past three months. She wanted to die at the farm. She told us she wasn't afraid, that she was ready. She told us her great life lesson: be nice—simple and profound. And even though she was dying, she thoughtfully scripted her death to make it easier for us.

This night was going to be okay.

I climbed up into the bed and shimmied over next to her.

I stroked her arm and held her hand. Her skin felt foreign, kind of thick and cool, not like Mom's skin. But I held on to her and talked to her.

I think tonight is going to be the night.

I know you're ready, but I sure hope you know how much I'm going to miss you.

We all love you like crazy, you know that?

I'm so proud of you, Mom.

I'm so glad you're my mom.

I don't know what time I finally fell asleep, but I know I stirred at least once and saw Sonia kneeling at Mom's side of the bed, crying as she talked to her. I didn't say anything and shut my eyes again because I didn't want to interrupt them.

I wondered if Mom would die when I was asleep, the same way Dad died. I wanted to believe that they chose to die when I was asleep, because I believed that's what they would have wanted, to not burden me, to comfort me somehow, even in their deaths.

At some point after midnight, Sonia's voice woke me up from where I was, curled up next to Mom, my pillow touching hers.

"Sarah, she's gone."

THE END OF SOMETHING

There is so much more I could tell you.

I could tell you about Joe coming over to the farm to wait for the people in the "meat wagon"—which is what we said even though we wondered if that was crass and awful and disrespectful—to come collect Mom's body. How we sat there in this strange limbo where we knew time was passing but it also wasn't, like we were suspended and watching as strangers entered the bedroom with a gurney to take her body away in the kind of thick, black bag you only see on detective shows when they go to the morgue to identify someone. And how they didn't really count all of the pills this time, which they are supposed to do every time to ensure we didn't overdose her, and instead we flushed them down the toilet and wondered if the cows out in the field might be high for the next week because we still didn't have city water at the farm.

I could tell you about the funeral, how even though it wasn't by invitation only as Mom originally suggested, the service was a beautiful reflection of who she was, and when we sang "Amazing Grace," I thought the roof of the church might break open to let such goodness and love out into the world.

I sat in the front row with Jane and Joe and their families, my DePauw girls and friends from New York in the rows behind us. I saw Camillus briefly before things started; I didn't know exactly where he was sitting, but I knew that I wanted to see him when the service ended. Our row got up to leave first. I scanned the crowded pews, found his eyes immediately, and felt him loaning me strength.

The reception at Bryan Place was packed with so many people, from "so many walks of life," as Mom would have said. Farmers, country clubbers, politicians, intellectuals, and everyone in between who wanted to be there. They all wanted to be in that place, on that day, to celebrate our collective, common-denominator love for Susan Gormley.

After the reception we went to the East End Cafe to drink beer, which felt like a tradition given we did the same thing when Dad died less than two years before, although I'm not sure two deaths are enough to constitute a tradition.

What you really need to know is that we had *fun*. We laughed and drank and cried and loved each other. I kept watching to make sure Jane and Joe weren't having meltdowns in a corner somewhere, and I remember Jane's eyes lighting up with one of her knowing glances when we realized one of the guests *might* have been more than a little overserved. Such things happen after a funeral, and the farmhouse was alive in celebration that night, likely the way it was when Mom and Dad threw their first parties there before Jane, Joe, and I even existed.

I was filled with wonder that we were there, together, the three little kids who had bounced around like jumping beans in the back of Mom's pickup truck as she sped down gravel roads, prompting more than one person to say, "You're going to kill those kids, Susan!"

But Mom didn't kill us.

Instead she was the best mom she could be, the woman who taught us how to live even when she showed us how to die.

TOMORROW WILL OCCUR

"Tomorrow will occur."

That's from a note Dad left for Mom on the kitchen table many years before. And now here I was, waking up in my childhood bedroom in the empty farmhouse wondering what I was going to do now that tomorrow was, in fact, here.

Mom was gone, the funeral was over, and my friends had flown home to New York, Chicago, Minneapolis, and Nashville and back to the rhythm of their daily lives. Life returned to normal for everyone else. But I had no normal, no schedule, and nothing to do for the first time in as long as I could remember. Just three months before, I had vowed to myself that I would intentionally do nothing for a *full year* to make sure I didn't fall back into gold-star chasing and making PowerPoint slides for the rest of my life.

I didn't know what to do, so I went downstairs to make coffee.

"Good morning, Sarah."

That text is how every day started when I didn't wake up next to Camillus.

I wondered how this thing between us might take a different shape, if our dynamic would change now that my role as caregiver was over. We had only been dating for two months, but when I thought about how easy it was between us and how natural it felt that Camillus was part of my days, doubt didn't have much room to spread. That part of my life felt so good and full. Sure, I had questions about his divorce and whether we were rushing into something, but unlike previous versions of myself—riddled with romantic analysis paralysis, expectations of doom and gloom, and questions around why it wouldn't work and what could go wrong—I just kept loving him.

"Good morning, Camillus."

***

I knew I would do some work on the farmhouse—small things like redoing hardwood floors and painting and not-small things like cleaning out fifty-plus years of stuff Mom and Dad stored in this corner or that. Joe would inherit the house and property, which we all agreed to years before Dad died. We didn't want the property to be sold or divided up, and Jane and I weren't as willing to take on the responsibility and enormous amount of work to maintain the farm.

Dad had been an estate attorney before he became a judge and knew these things should be discussed and agreed upon before parents die to avoid the ugliness that seems to happen far too often in families. Our hope was that Joe and his family would move in and keep the place alive with the next generation. We rented a huge dumpster, which sat over at the church, and I would proudly count the bags of trash I learned to heave up and over from the truck bed in one smooth motion. I thought perhaps there should be a new Olympic sport dedicated to this talent. More than once, Joe climbed into the dumpster to retrieve items he didn't believe should be thrown out, like coasters Dad received in a golf tournament or some part of a grill that probably hadn't been used in seventeen years, which I teased him about mercilessly.

The cleaning lady emptied out Mom's medicine cabinet but left one last can of Copenhagen and her last bottle of Chanel No. 5, which is the perfume I've worn every day since she died.

I planned to travel. I took trips to New York, Chicago, Maine, Boston, Montauk, and Nashville. I wanted to visit friends where they lived, spend time with them in their homes, and *not* talk about Mom's death and instead talk about their kids' baseball games, how hot it was outside, and where we might go for dinner. I helped Tippett make snow cones at a school carnival in Glenview, Illinois, pouring just the right amount of flavored bright orange or red onto the mound of crushed ice, which felt like the best thing I'd accomplished in years.

I noticed that not one of my friends seemed to miss me talking about work, getting up to take calls, or apologizing again about sending *just one last* email from the table, stressed about whether I was going to be promoted, whether I was getting the raise, or how so-and-so or such-and-such was making it impossible to do the job I was hired to do.

Although they didn't say so explicitly, I suspected they preferred this unemployed version of me, and if I'd asked, I'm certain they would have agreed that the corporate-climbing me was their least favorite side of me.

Camillus and I went for lots and lots of drives. Sometimes we got up before sunrise, took our coffee, and hit the dirt roads we knew would take us to the top of a hill for the best view. Other times, we set out with the goal of finding the best little dive bar in whatever town we happened upon when a cold Miller Lite started to sound good.

We pulled off a country highway so I could talk to a pair of horses in a field one afternoon. I started crying, and when Camillus asked me what was wrong, I told him I hadn't known it was possible to be so happy and so sad at the same time, that I thought there should be a better word for what my friend Shawna called "double-dip" emotions, a term she learned from a children's book. I loved to reach my left arm over and stroke the back of his neck when he was driving. He later admitted that it tickled and he actually couldn't stand the feeling, but he never said anything because he knew how it comforted me.

***

I started writing again, sometimes when the emotion was only grief, on days when the pain felt like too much, like there was no way happiness was going to come back in.

I talked to David every Tuesday about grief and how to live with unknowns. We revisited regular topics about being angry when our needs aren't met, and how nobody *makes* you feel something—that you feel the way you feel because of how you are wired—and how difficult change can be even when it's for the better.

We kept swimming around the pond, dipping down and coming back up, paddling around the same circles, but every lap slightly different from the one before. We kept going, and I recognized myself more every day.

ORPHAN CHILD

Your parents
do not tell you
how this will be.
They are not there to tell you.
Because they are dead.
Both of them.
It's Father's Day, and you're driving
on Route 16, toward home.
But you know, with the weight of for sure,
forever, for certain, certainty,
that home will never be home again.
Because they are dead.
Both of them.
And you're the saddest orphan
you've ever met.
Which is a fine line
in a book of poetry
filed under *grief*
on a dusty shelf in the back of the bookstore
nobody visits.
But the line doesn't tell the pain.
Doesn't describe the sharp fingers
that dig into the bottom of your heart,

peeling upward only to meet
the suffocating hot tears
and thick snot
that keep coming, months and months later.
You sit in this suffering
until you are ready.
Until you are ready to tell the world
I am an orphan child.
Did I lose them or did they lose me?
Which orphan would I rather be?

OCTOBER, LATER THAT YEAR

The sky was a brilliant blue on one of those perfect fall days, still warm but not hot, the sun hanging on for a few more minutes of summer.

Camillus and I were out for a buggy ride, driving through the tall grass in the hayfield and then down next to the power line that led to Salt Creek, which we'd cross at a shallow point before heading up the driveway.

He slowed down and told me he had a question for me, something he'd never asked but was curious about.

"Well, I happen to be taking questions, Camillus," I said. "Go ahead."

I loved that we had been dating for ten months, which was not only a record for me but long enough to have inside jokes, little codes between us that reminded us we were together, like saying each other's names more than necessary and "taking questions," which he had used the first time he picked me up to go buy a mattress.

"What's your favorite spot on the farm?"

I had never thought about this before, even after being so connected to the land for more than forty years.

"I really don't know that I have a favorite spot, which is weird," I said. "I guess I just love the whole place."

"Huh." He kind of shrugged his shoulders and nodded and drove on.

And then, as if his simple question had conjured a revelation, I knew the real answer. The tears started coming in a wave of emotion that surprised me even though I had become quite the crier since Mom died. Camillus hated seeing me cry. He stopped the buggy, turned toward me, and put his hands on my shoulders.

"Oh no," he said. "Please don't cry. I didn't mean to upset you."

But I wasn't upset. I was happy. All of a sudden I was nine years old again, galloping on my horse up a narrow trail as we often did on the way back to the barn. Frosty knew this route meant it was time for grain or hay and usually sped up on the last little turn to the right. Somehow my leg grazed a tree, catching the stirrup strap, and I flew off as Frosty continued to the barn.

I was stunned when I hit the ground and checked my arms and legs to see if anything was broken. I wasn't hurt so I walked to the barn, took off her bridle and saddle, and gave her some grain. I was probably scolding her about leaving me on the trail when I noticed one of the stirrups had come off during my fall. I'm not sure if they saw the riderless horse first or me walking down the hill horseless, but Mom and Dad came out to the barn to see if I was okay. I told them I was fine, but I'd lost a stirrup and needed to go find it.

The three of us walked back up to the trail and found it off to the side near a patch of thornbushes I was glad I didn't land in. I assumed we would go back to the house because I knew they were supposed to be going to a party at the country club that night and probably had to get ready. I asked them about it, and Dad said they weren't going, which I guessed must have been because they were worried about me somehow. What I hadn't yet known was that Dad was in renal failure and he was going to need a kidney transplant as soon as possible.

Dad sat down on the hill facing the house, about midway down from the top, so that we could just see the house across the field. After Mom sat down, I squeezed in between them, close enough that I could feel their arms and legs pressing into mine, as if we were one entity. I don't know how long we sat there or what we talked about. But I remember laughing. And I remember thinking this was a special moment, that I was a lucky girl to be sitting there like that, the three of us on a hillside.

I explained all of this to Camillus.

"That spot on the hill is my favorite place on the farm, but I hadn't thought about it until you asked me just now," I told him.

Camillus hugged me so tight that I felt his heart beating.

We continued down the hill and across Salt Creek.

I thought we would go up to the house, but he drove past the driveway, and when he turned left, I realized he was taking us up the same trail from that day so many years ago. I looked over at Camillus, squeezed his leg, and smiled, undone by this small gesture that told me everything about the man I loved. This moment mattered to him because it mattered to me.

We drove up to where the trees started to narrow, and I tried to guess which one was my tree from that day.

We emerged from the woods near the spot on the hillside.

I saw myself sitting there as a little girl with my short hair and boys' Levi's, a little sweaty, my fingers dirty from clenching on to Frosty's mane as we galloped. I could feel Dad's arm around my shoulders and hear Mom's laugh as she threw her head back. Part of me wanted to stay there with them, to feel them loving me again.

But I also wanted to come back, to be me sharing this moment with Camillus.

Here I was, forty-six, both my parents dead. I was an adult orphan. I had no job and no idea what job would be next. I had no home of my own and no idea where my next home would be. And yet, I was smiling. The sun hit my face, my eyes the bright blue they become after I've been crying. I was in a mud-covered buggy sitting next to a kind and beautiful man whose love opened parts of my head and heart I didn't know existed. The biggest decision I had to make at the moment was what to have for dinner. I would figure that out and then figure out the next thing because I was okay.

I was better than okay.

Right then, I knew who I was and who I was meant to be.

My life had been waiting for me all along.

As we drove toward the house and watched the reluctant sun begin to set, I realized I knew something else.

I was ready to leave the farm.

EPILOGUE

Some people say the book will tell you when it's time to end it. "You'll just know," these people who know such things say. But I'm not sure I know how to end this story, because there is so much more I could tell you.

I could tell you about how Mom's enormous wooden bowl from the farm now sits on my kitchen counter in the first home I've ever owned.

I might tell you about opening an art gallery, which is something I've dreamed about since college.

I'd definitely tell you about Camillus. How he makes the best egg sandwiches for breakfast, talks to the little succulents in his kitchen window, and complains that I'm a hot sleeper. I'd wonder about what not to share, too, and decide to keep some things just for us, because I'm learning that the intimacy between us is a gift I'm not ready to give away. I will tell you that when we go for drives in his truck, I refrain from touching the back of his neck even though I really, really want to sometimes.

All of these things are important to me, but they aren't really what you need to know.

***

What I want you to know is that my life changed in ways I never could have fathomed.

I hated myself and thought I would never escape the running tape that told me I wasn't enough, that I was a piece of shit, that I wasn't worthy. I thought the running tape would define me more than any gold star ever could. I thought the self-loathing was who I *was* rather than the thing I had to *figure out*, the thing I had to work through to get to the good thing.

Me. I'm the good thing. Or at least *a* good thing.

And I still can't believe how lucky I am that I figured it out—how profound and weird and strange and scary it is to live in this new way— but I'm never going back and not letting the pain back in because fuck that shit. I lived there for thirty-five years, and that wasted pain doesn't get one more day of me. Or maybe the pain wasn't wasted, because you know what? Here I am. Here I fucking am. Maybe the pain and all three parts of the Venn diagram, including heredity and environment and the part that is uniquely me, and that first email to David and my stubborn insistence that I wanted and deserved more for my life than all of the exhaustive chasing actually helped. Maybe the universe aligns itself just for us sometimes, or maybe we just believe it does because how else does it make sense that you can fall wildly, madly in love with the kindest man you've ever met while your mom is dying? How the fuck does that happen? Because it can't be what the self-help gurus up on stage tell you—that love will happen when you're ready. But what if they are right? And how do we know we're ready or not ready or when to do the work or even start the work or know what lever to pull first and how to start taking a deep breath when you need a fucking break and just want to exhale but you have to keep going, just keep going? And then one Thursday afternoon when you're pulling away from a gas station when you're forty-seven years old you find yourself weeping over the steering wheel because you think your heart might explode with so much gratitude that this is your life and you don't know how you got so fucking lucky and you think you're a smart girl who likes to really understand things with logic but sometimes it's okay to say *I do not know*—not entirely anyway and definitely not with any certainty because life is not about order—and no matter how hard I try, maybe I'll never know how to write about the thing that is so much harder to explain than to feel.

I do not know.

There is no formula.

The order of things will change.

TWO YEARS PASS

(THAT'S WHAT A MOVIE SCREEN WOULD SAY RIGHT NOW.)

RUSSIAN DOLLS, OR WHY THE FIRST ENDING WASN'T REALLY THE END

"How's the book coming?" friends asked me.

I had told everyone I was writing a memoir when I started. And I was writing a memoir. I decided in August 2020 to write this thing, and I had what I thought was a great manuscript finished by August 2021. HOORAY! Let's pick out the actress who will play me in the movie. Jennifer Lawrence, of course, permitting that the inevitable publishing and production delays allow her to age closer to my age in the book.

"I don't really know," I told them. "I've been stuck." I had been stuck for almost two years. I would do nothing for months, then try to dig in again and run out of steam, frustrated by what felt like a lack of progress. "Turns out editing a manuscript is way fucking harder than writing the first draft." I say "way fucking harder" every time, as if I want even nonwriters to understand that it is *way fucking harder.*

Writing is magic. Look at me: I have ideas, and I put words down on paper in a rhythm that can make you laugh or cry, and sometimes both. I'm talented. I'm an artist. I'm a writer. I love the writing part. Editing is much fucking harder. Editing is like cleaning out the basement after your parents die. It's sad and awful and painful, and I don't want to do it, not for one more second. Because wasn't this stuff good enough to hold on to at some point? Like the wooden toy horse on wheels down there that I loved? Now I'm supposed to throw it away? Editing means cutting out and discarding pages of my life to keep the real estate nice and tidy for the new inhabitant, the better manuscript. Getting rid of certain things to make the next version better. Hard as hell. And kind of like life, if you want to get all deep about things.

Yuck. But I did the work. I cut sixty-eight pages. Gold stars.

It's all there, and the edited version is much better, tighter than the first draft, narrowed down to a period of time just as two agents recommended after they read the first draft. The action takes place over my year at the farm, leaving my career, meeting Camillus, and Mom dying. And therapy. Don't forget the emotional healing. Another hooray for healing. It's all there, and you already know this because you just read that part. The edited version came in too short for a book, and I don't know if a *memoirella* is even a thing.

Maybe it's fear of failure, or the fear that I won't get a book deal. Or maybe I'm lazy. Nah. I'm a lot of things and can procrastinate sometimes, but I'm not lazy. My best guess is I'm afraid I won't know where the story ends. The year at the farm feels far away now, and the distance in the rearview mirror makes it easier to see what happened, in what order.

I lived at the family farm for a year. Important things happened. My life changed in profound ways. The end. Right? But I'm writing this part in 2023, and life is still happening. There are more things I want to tell you. Things are happening now because of what happened before, because of the order. More poems, for instance. You want more of those, right?

I feel like the fattest outer layer in a set of Russian stacking dolls. And the Sarah protagonist—the narrator of the feel-good memoir, the one who was finally ready to leave the farm? She's like four entire dolls ago in the order of things, and the set keeps getting bigger because my life keeps getting bigger. Life gets fatter, but the manuscript needs to get leaner; how's that for a mind fuck? A dear friend of mine was once informed that she was "the skinny fat girl"—by a man, of course, who thought it was a compliment. Said man was then a closeted gay man, so maybe we should forgive him? But the term works for what I'm giving you now, my skinny-fat-girl end of a memoir.

A FEW WORDS ON MOM

This was never supposed to be a book about Mom. Yes, it's a book that includes a lot about my relationship with her, and the arc takes place as she lay dying (I see you, William Faulkner): grief and untangling and becoming the me who is separate from her. There likely are at least four more books I could write chronicling my relationship with her, or even a more journalistic book entirely about her life.

But here's the thing: last week I started writing an essay about how I seem to be bringing artists into my life who remind me of her. *Assembling* might be the better word, but I felt as if I was collecting them, almost like art, to become part of my life. I knew the essay would be good, profound even, because I was entirely unaware of the collecting until I heard one of the women say something, and suddenly it was as if Mom was right there on her blue sofa uttering the exact words. Christiane's turn of phrase, Sharon's exuberance, and Susanne's style. Each one of them carries qualities of Mom I've started to see clearly. I started outlining and writing and thinking about where I might submit this essay-to-be, and then it hit me: I don't really want to write about Mom anymore. I don't care how good the essay will be.

There, I said it. I didn't want to write that essay (although I'm not a quitter, so you're going to read it pretty soon) because I wanted to get back to finishing this memoir. And even though her presence and influence are undeniable, the rest of this story is not about Mom; the rest of the story—the whole story in fact—is about me and the strange and beautiful life I've created. The rest of the story is about how we're always becoming the largest Russian doll. What happens to us—and the life we create, edit, and revise for ourselves—keeps changing. As soon as you write it, it can be erased, but every experience influences the next, and the doll keeps getting bigger.

BLACK HOUSES

Let me show you my home. I've had many addresses in my life but only one house with my name on the deed. Or is it a title? There's a piece of paper in Camillus's safe—I lose things all of the time, so his safe holds important things an adult should not lose—that shows that I own this little black farmhouse in the city, tucked away on a narrow brick street in Italian Village.

The late afternoon light is shining through the windows into the living room with the long and deep sofa I bought when I moved to San Francisco, where I had an enormous living room and made so much money I could buy big, fancy sofas to help fill up my life.

Behind the sofa is the first painting I ever owned, the one Grandma Cameron bought for me when I graduated from DePauw and is still my favorite in the collection that spreads from room to room. Grandma and I didn't know I'd end up opening the art gallery twenty-five years later. That painting greets me every time I walk in the room, a reminder of where I am and where I came from. Little Edie Beale is on the sofa, grooming herself near a green velvet pillow and meowing at me to pay attention to her.

There's a huge wooden bowl on the kitchen island. Mom bought it at an antique store and filled it with salads for twenty-five people when they had summer parties at the farm. The bowl is one of the few things I took from the farm after she died, and now it sits on the counter at my home.

My home.

Home.

I've lived in great cities, and I've lived in gorgeous apartments. But until now, I've only ever called one place "home," and that was the farm. When you rent, you are free. You can come, and you can go. No leaking roof or broken washing machine is your burden. Other people take care of such things. When Mom got sick, I felt so relieved and so smart that I could be home in mere weeks without having to worry about selling a house.

I knew this house would become my home the minute I put my hand on the old wooden door that had a rickety knob and the original house number hand stenciled in chipped gold on the transom above, and I knew I would paint it black. It feels like the home of the girl who grew up on the farm and the young woman who went to New York City. It feels like the home of the barefoot little girl playing down by Salt Creek who became the woman who owns an art gallery.

***

"I've been painting houses for thirty years, but I've never painted one black."

"I've only seen one black house before . . . but I sure didn't paint it—it was an old farmhouse out there on Clay Pike, in Chandlersville."

I overheard Greg and Steve's banter, two men I'd never met before, part of the crew at my new house, my little farmhouse in Columbus, Ohio. It's the first house I've ever owned, and while it's just an hour west of the farm, the path that took me away and then brought me back to Ohio can't really be measured in miles. My coming home is still something that doesn't make sense on any map beyond the complicated navigation of the human heart.

"Guess what, Steve? That black farmhouse out in Chandlersville you saw? That's the house I grew up in!"

I'm not the first Gormley woman to paint a house black.

I was around twelve when Gary Okey showed up far too early to paint one summer morning. I awoke to the ladders and scaffolding banging out in the front yard. My bedroom spanned the entire width of the house, with huge windows that opened in like doors. When I popped up in bed, there was Gary, looking at me through the warped and worn screen with a knowing grin spread out above his pointy chin.

"I'd say it's about time for you to be out of bed, isn't it, Sarah?"

I hadn't left for summer camp yet. I didn't think Gary was nearly as funny as he did, even though I always knew he was a good man. He wasn't just a painter. He was one of our neighbors, a farmer who lived on Wolf Run Road about three miles away, which didn't make him our closest neighbor, but in Chandlersville, among farmers, it was close enough. Neighbors were the people you trusted most, who you could call in the middle of the night when a cow was sick or when the truck was stuck in a snowbank at the end of your long driveway.

Gary generally painted my parents' house when he decided it needed to be painted, without even asking them. He just showed up in his white truck with all of the canvas drop cloths and a metal lunch bucket to settle in for the day. He had originally told Mom he wasn't going to paint her house black—he refused. The house had been the same Gary-approved Williamsburg blue-gray with brown trim forever, and Gary liked it that way.

"I'm pretty sure I can find another painter who would paint the damn house whatever color I want!" Mom told him, a not-so-subtle reminder that even though he was a neighbor, she was paying him to do a job.

Gary painted the house black.

More than thirty years later, the farmhouse was still black. Shortly after Mom died, it seemed like a good idea to refresh some of the interior, especially the kitchen. I called Gary, who was by then nearly eighty. He and his wife, like all of our neighbors, were mourning Mom's death. I thought about how different it felt for them to drive down Clay Pike knowing she was gone.

Gary showed up unannounced a week or so later, far too early on a Monday morning. He carried his ladders and brought in the canvas drop cloths and walked more stiffly than he did so many summers ago when he woke me up that morning when I was a girl. That first day, we sat at the kitchen table as he ate his lunch out of the same metal lunch bucket, and he told me the story about Mom insisting that she wanted a black house.

"She was a woman who knew what she wanted," he said as he took a bite out of the same sandwich I imagined he had been eating for more than forty years.

HOW THE ART THING STARTED

I was completely hungover, and the supersize McDonald's Coke that Dad brought to the sorority house wasn't much help. Barbara Kingsolver was our commencement speaker, and the Phi Beta Kappa (gold stars!) English literature nerd in me was thrilled by the thought of hearing her talk.

Graduation started at eleven on the lawn near Meharry Hall, the oldest building on DePauw's campus. In the convoluted way that life happens, I was invited to deliver the class address at our twenty-fifth class reunion in Meharry Hall partly because Grandma Cameron bought me a painting the morning I graduated. We'll get to that.

The day was sticky, and families were already filling in the rows of plastic folding chairs in the shade when Mom, Dad, Grandma, and I walked into Emison Art Center. I wanted to show them a painting by my classmate Matt Wenc, a studio art major from Chicago. Matt played soccer and was known to walk in his sleep, but I didn't know him beyond his friendly "Hey, Gorms, how's it going?" when we passed each other on the North Quad. I didn't own any other pieces of art, although I cherished my *Mount Fuji and Flowers* David Hockney print from the Metropolitan Museum of Art I'd had since high school. The farmhouse didn't have a lot of art in it, either, aside from some old needlepoint samplers and a couple of pieces my brother and sister painted as kids, the kind of things parents frame and then wonder how long they have to keep.

I'd gone to the senior art show and couldn't stop thinking about the two large pieces Matt painted. I learned that together, two paintings were called a diptych—which meant they were to be seen together—although he put individual prices on each one just in case. The one I wanted and hoped Grandma Cameron might buy for me as a graduation gift was full of bright, warm colors—oranges, reds, and yellows. Although it was abstract, he told my roommate and me that it was inspired by a trip he took to Rome. The sister painting was much cooler, mainly whites and blues, an intentional contrast. I remember thinking that together, the paintings might represent the array of emotions a person can carry simultaneously, and looking back, I find it surprising I was drawn to the one with more heat. The price was $500, and I have to believe Matt didn't actually anticipate it would sell.

I couldn't wait to show Grandma, who had asked me the last time I was home what I wanted for my graduation gift. The four of us were alone in the building, a square limestone structure that felt more like a government building than an art gallery.

"This is the painting," I said, thinking my enthusiasm would prompt a reaction from the woman whose Revlon-lipsticked lips typically stayed pressed together in a sharp line. She wasn't mean per se; she was just chillier than your made-for-TV grandma.

"Well, I don't know what it is," she said, in a tone more than slightly dismissive, "but if you really want it, I am happy to buy it for you."

I smiled at her. I was her youngest grandchild, and I knew she was proud of me even if she thought I was a little "progressive" for a girl from Ohio, what with my poetry writing, hankering to move to New York City, and desire to own *real* art.

Out of the corner of my eye, I saw Matt Wenc and his mother walk in. I was surprised to see him and wondered if Grandma thought we might have planned this to encourage the sale. I don't remember now, but I don't think I even told Matt that I wanted the painting much less planned for our chance encounter.

"Matt, I can't believe you're here. These are my parents, and this is my Grandma Cameron. She might buy your painting for me."

Matt's eyes widened. We all stood there in silence, awkward given that Matt and I weren't really close friends and this would be the only point in time these six people would be in the same room.

"Well, let's do this so I can get a seat in the shade before the ceremony starts."

Grandma took Matt by the arm and steered him to a corner of the room. It's entirely possible she was wearing white gloves, which seems unbelievable today, but that's the kind of woman she was. She opened her black patent-leather pocketbook, the rectangular kind with a mouth that opens wide, and pulled out a roll of cash with a rubber band around the middle because she was also that kind of woman. I could tell she asked Matt how much the painting cost, and then watched as she counted off five one-hundred-dollar bills. Matt seemed a little speechless as a smile spread across his face.

In May 1994, Grandma Cameron and Matt Wenc shook hands, and I became the owner of a real piece of art.

Twenty-five years later, I opened Sarah Gormley Gallery.

AN ART GALLERY IN REVERSE CHRONOLOGICAL ORDER

September 2023

Sarah Gormley Gallery (SGG) is voted the best gallery in Columbus, Ohio, by the readers of *Columbus Monthly*. The margin was quite small, and I think Camillus's family members may have voted twice, but I'm proud of myself, and my heart swells every time I walk into the gallery.

September 2022

SGG moves downtown, into a larger space with poured-concrete floors, high ceilings, and perfect lighting. Four massive wooden doors mark the front entrance. When people see the new space, they almost always say, "This feels just like a New York gallery," and I nod, then smile and say, "But it's not, you're in a Columbus gallery." And every time, I think about the man in New York City from so many years before who helped determine the ethos of SGG—that art can be a source of joy for everyone, but no assholes allowed.

April 2019

SGG opens, originally planned as a pop-up gallery to get it out of my system. I built a website and designed a logo and quickly realized this wasn't just an experiment, even though I know that I'm allowing myself to make up this part of my career as I go along. And it turns out the least-planned, least-thought-out job I've had is the most interesting and rewarding thing I've ever done, and I haven't even created a single PowerPoint slide.

October 2015

I buy myself a painting by David Kramer called *Marketer's Dream*, which makes fun of the marketing profession, when I take the big marketing job with Adobe. In the painting, a woman who looks like a pinup girl tilts her head and below her a quote reads "I don't care what they are selling, I want it anyway. I am a marketer's dream." My art collection is a visual story of my life, each painting chosen at a particular point in time, a marker of emotional growth, a part of some order I couldn't see at the time.

June 1999

I stop by a gallery on the Upper East Side of Manhattan, where I now live, to ask if they can recommend somebody to help hang art in my studio apartment. I only own a few pieces, but I know enough to hire an expert when it comes to installing. Mister Gallery Asshole looks me up and down and asks if I have a "sizable" collection with a thick level of condescension. I assure him I do not have a "sizable" collection but suggest that an art installer is likely paid by the hour so perhaps the installer should decide if my collection is *sizable* enough. The installer shows up the next day, and I remain his client my entire sixteen years in New York. Though I don't refer to myself as one, I'm already an art collector.

May 1994

Grandma Cameron gives me my first piece of art when I graduate from DePauw. I told you this part already.

THANKSGIVING BREAKFAST

You were in the kitchen
frying bacon for egg sandwiches
when my tears started pooling up
from the bottom, the way water fills a spoon.
You said something about me not washing
my coffee cup, teasing with
the sweet snark of morning routine
but couldn't see my face
because my back was to you.
This was my fourth Thanksgiving without
    parents.
No living parents, that is.
I understand they're still my parents and will be
every Thanksgiving to come.
Grief finds me like this sometimes,
sneaks into the room the way my cat curls
around my ankles, and I know it's her because
I know the feeling all too well.
I don't want you to see me crying
because it's been four years
and your father died in August.
I think you deserve
all of the grief servings today.

When I don't respond
you walk over to the table.
I hear your steps on the stone floor
and feel your flannel shirt brush my arm
before I turn my head
to let you see me.
Something passes between us
for which there is no word.
I am hungry, but I am full.

BREAKFAST IN A DINER WE DON'T NORMALLY FREQUENT

The waitress had just delivered our omelets when Camillus put his knife and fork down like a punctuation mark. Like he had something to tell me. "I talked to my boss on Friday, and they're planning to make changes to the product lineup."

He has worked for the same company for nearly fifteen years, making top salesman every year—or at least that's how I saw it. He made them a shit ton of money, which I knew meant he would be fine regardless of what changed. I loved being out of the corporate world, but I missed the camaraderie and helping colleagues navigate the inevitable minefield of politics and personalities.

"Okay, so what do you think that means for you?"

"I'm actually pretty worried. I've been talking less with the CEO and more with his son who will be taking over—"

"BUT YOU'RE THE TOP SALESPERSON!" I interrupted, so full of confidence for him that I didn't want doubt to enter his mind. "Camillus, you've been there so long and made them so much money, there's no way—"

"Can I finish?" His voice was firm, and I squirmed in my seat like a little kid being scolded.

"I'm starting to think it's probably time for me to start looking at new things, and I worry about giving up my flexibility with the kids' schedules—"

"But you can fix this! Just figure out what the new product line is, and tell them you want six months to grow that part of the business, which I know you can do."

"SARAH!" He was loud enough that other customers looked. "Just stop. Can you please not try to problem solve this one? I just want you to listen right now."

I felt my face turn red and hot, tears filling up past the bottom lid, anger suddenly spreading through my limbs.

"I'm so sorry for trying to be fucking helpful," I hissed, seething. "Sorry about supporting you. Would you prefer I doubt you and make you feel worse—is that what you want?"

"Are you kidding me right now? What are you talking about?"

"I'm talking about you not valuing my opinion. That's pretty clear, and I've had some experience in the real world, you know. I happen to know things other than how to barely make an art gallery succeed." I still carried some defensiveness after leaving the corporate career I'd toiled in for twenty-five years—still wanted credit for my success somehow.

"No, that's not what I'm saying, and I do value your opinion or we wouldn't be dating. Why are you making this about you?"

"You just told me to shut up. Wasn't that about me? Better yet, when in the hell is it going to be about me? We've been together five years, so why don't you tell me when my opinion starts to count, Camillus?"

I added his name at the end because we were affectionate name callers—we loved saying each other's names—and I knew that saying it in a heated moment would be a special zinger. I wanted to hurt him the way he hurt me, and the adrenaline carried me out of the diner just as quickly as I'd allowed the anger to take over my body.

I was shaking when I got to the parking lot, and ordered a Lyft. I didn't even turn around to look for him, because I knew Camillus wasn't coming after me.

I think about that morning, that scene, and how it unfolded all of the time.

Except that is not what happened.

***

The conversation started the same, with Camillus telling me about the changes in the product lineup, me interrupting him, and then him asking me not to problem solve.

"SARAH!" He was loud enough that other customers looked. "Just stop. Can you please not try to problem solve this one? I just want you to listen right now."

I felt my face turn red and hot, tears filling up past the bottom lid.

Camillus rarely raises his voice or cuts me off, and he knows I hate yelling. I felt the anger cells spreading, the mitosis of rage starting deep down, and sat on my hands to keep myself from leading with a gesture, not letting my body get ahead of my heart. Deep breath. Bite of omelet. Look at him. Look at this man across from you. I thought about how often he tells me he appreciates me, how he puts his hands on my shoulders and makes me look into his eyes when he tells me. I thought about how he actively tries not to hurt me.

Most of all, I thought about how really, really difficult it is for me to shut the fuck up sometimes.

I nodded so Camillus knew I heard him. I ate my omelet as he talked. I was listening, but all the while, as if on one of the television screens above the bar, I saw the other version of the scene playing out. I saw what would have happened if I let the younger, untherapied me— the insecure me who would have gotten defensive and insisted on being heard—react. I watched her storm out into the parking lot in a dramatic exit, saw the tears, and heard snippets of the ensuing phone call to Nancy about what an asshole he had been.

I asked myself if the other version of me got what she wanted. I thought about telling Camillus about the other scene, how I still felt the instincts of my previous self, and how I get defensive and combative when I let my insecurities lead. I thought about all of these things and decided I didn't need to say another thing, at least not that morning, not in that diner.

Instead, I simply let Camillus talk. And I let myself appreciate being with a man who knows how to ask for what he needs. Most of all, I relished the feeling of being somebody's chosen audience.

THERAPY ABOUT THE DINER

"Seriously, I don't know how anybody stays married or in a relationship, especially if they don't have children keeping them motivated to keep trying. This shit is fucking hard."

Being in a relationship with Camillus is fascinating on many levels, and I continue to be amazed by how quickly things can unravel if just one of the two people in *any* relationship is emotionally off, not to mention both people at the same time. After the nonfight that morning, I kept thinking about calibration, or what I thought calibration was—how you make tiny adjustments to get back to healthy, functioning levels. I spent a lot of time working on my own calibration and wondered if other people have to try so hard to maintain themselves or if at some point it all just comes naturally.

In my session with David the Tuesday morning after the diner scene, I told him about how I watched the previous version of myself have a meltdown, possibly one that would have ended the best relationship I've ever been in. I was proud of myself and wanted David to see how far I'd come.

"Good for you," he said. "Sounds as if you handled that very well."

I was in the blue swivel chair in my living room, where I usually sat for our phone sessions, and I knew he had more to say—something constructive, no doubt.

"Do you really think that the two of you would have broken up if you had walked out?"

I paused longer than normal and made that *woooooollllll* sound that admitted I hadn't thought about other scenarios. David went on to suggest that the breakup conclusion sounded extreme and not very modulated. There it was: Modulation is never going to be my strong suit. I'm always working on fucking modulation, keeping perspective, not assuming the worst.

"We should talk about why you don't have more belief in the strength of the container."

I had no idea what David meant.

"Like a shipping container?" It's amazing he doesn't fire me. I know I'm one of his success stories (gold stars!), but sometimes I swear he thinks I regress years in a single session.

"Not exactly. It's more of a metaphor about trusting that the container of your relationship can support what you're feeling and how you express what you're feeling to the person you love."

"I seriously think Camillus would have broken up with me if I'd gone with Sarah number one that day."

"I'm not sure I agree with you. I'm impressed that you managed to control your initial anger that morning, but I think you are too cautious about sharing how you feel with him sometimes. Do you really think he would have ended what you have with each other because of one fight, even if you acted 'batshit crazy,' to put it in your words?"

I had been so proud of myself and how far I'd come that I wasn't ready for even more . . . *growth*. There was always more to learn.

"Well, I don't know. I think he has, like, zero tolerance for any bullshit. Even with me."

"*Even* with you? You're not some random person. You are Sarah, and what you have together is beautiful. He *chose* you."

David was right. Again. I took a deep breath and reset. Becoming and being emotionally healthy is exhausting. Like, endless-marathon exhausting. But the payoff is everything. I took another look at the ending of the first diner scene, and you know what? I quickly realized that Camillus wouldn't have broken up with me.

Camillus would have come out to the parking lot and made a joke about this being the only time he'd seen me leave half an omelet uneaten, anywhere. He would have wrapped me up in his arms and let me cry. Then he would have asked me emphatically to stop crying because he hates seeing me cry. When we got back inside, he would have said, "Sarah, I want to tell you about something going on at work, and I'm asking you to listen," with a twinkle in his eye that would bring us back. He would reset us. Camillus would have helped me handle me, and I would have let him.

Now, do I need to go back and revise the diner scene I wrote? The order of things just changed again.

This shit is fucking hard, people. Mind your containers.

THIS MORNING AT THE GIANT EAGLE IN GRANDVIEW

I bought a container of dates,
not able to recall the last time
I'd tasted one.
I pried back the clear plastic lid
and brought the wrinkled fruit to my mouth,
biting into the sweet flesh
but forgetting about the pit,
which stayed lodged in my cheek
through the cereal
and canned good aisles.

I thought about the famous poem
with the plums from the icebox
and felt nostalgic for a memory
that wasn't mine.

Then I realized that dates are not plums
and tucked the pit into the pocket
of my boyfriend's button-down.

I wear his shirt like a note he's left for me.

HIGHWAY SIGNS

Christiane was wearing a blue sleeveless housedress with tiny pink and yellow flowers, the kind of dress a woman of her refinement definitely wouldn't wear out to dinner or even to the grocery store. She's one of the artists I represent, and I was visiting her to talk about an upcoming show at the gallery. She is French, which adds an air of elegance to her eighty-five years, a number that seems to surprise her. She has twin daughters, but I try to check in on her regularly. She lives alone aside from her black cat, who stays curled up on the sofa when I visit.

She tells me that she's struggling to finish a series for the next show. "I try to paint every day, but sometimes it's difficult for me. I have to make breakfast and clean up the kitchen and then make sure to take care of the garden. And I have to nap. I am finding that I am just so tired," Christiane said, letting her arms fall down into her lap, punctuating the word "tired."

I don't know if it was the lilt of her voice or the specific way her hands were positioned, palms up, but for a brief moment, and for the first time in the four years since I've known Christiane, I saw Mom. The moment made me pause, almost gasp. Was this emotional déjà vu? I knew she was Christiane and not my mother, of course, but there was something about her, or in her, that was like Mom.

I got in the car and couldn't shake what had just happened, the significance not lost on me as I drove back home. Then, all of a sudden, I saw the faces of two other older women I've met in the years since Mom died. It felt as if the moment with Christiane uncovered something I'd not yet realized: I was surrounded by women who reminded me of Mom. With Christiane, it's her elegant acceptance of her age and her exhaustion—her admission of being *just so tired*.

Sharon owns an art gallery and is beloved by everyone who knows her. Always smiling, she's stylish the way a woman who collects antiques is stylish: the perfect gold signet ring, a cashmere scarf casually tied about her neck. I first met with her when I was contemplating opening SGG, and even though she'd just met me, she didn't hesitate: "Of course you can do it! You'll figure it out, and it's going to be wonderful." Now, to be clear, Mom wasn't always that supportive of me—and if she was still alive, she might wonder if I was ever going to get a *real* job again—but she thrived on counseling others who were in the midst of making life decisions. She had an uncanny way of breaking through bullshit. Sharon loaned me her confidence and continues to do so every time I ask for guidance. The thing that most reminds me of Mom is how her face lights up when she throws her arms up in the air to give me a hug every time she sees me.

Susanne is a firecracker. Having finished her master's degree at seventy-four, she's one of SGG's top-selling artists, and people love her as a person just as much as they love her vibrant, abstract floral paintings. On top of that, she has a shock of white hair and is one of the most stylish women in Columbus. I realized Susanne is Mom too. The white hair, the fuck-it-I'm-doing-it! attitude, the way she walks into a room. Mom had a long navy Donna Karan coatdress I borrowed twice and wish I still owned today given its timeless design. Unfortunately, Mom donated the dress before I could claim it for my closet. One day I met Susanne for lunch to talk about her next show. She walked in wearing a navy Donna Karan jacket, and I got goose bumps because I could see Mom's physical frame in Susanne.

Yes, I recognized the similar jacket, but I didn't yet realize this wasn't all coincidence: I was collecting women who carried elements of Mom. In her absence, I'd found a way to hold on to the things I most loved about her, keeping her alive and with me through them. When I talked to David about it, he didn't seem at all surprised, but we both agreed that this insight into self-awareness earned me a gold star in therapy, one of the stars I continue to seek after ten years of meeting with him weekly. Today, however, I recognize when I earn one, and let myself enjoy minor and major accomplishments, all the while making fun of myself for still wanting the stars.

***

Months later, I drove to the museum in Canton, Ohio, to meet with an artist named Amy Pleasant. Yes, that's her name. She lives outside Seattle now but grew up in a small town not far from mine. Her current body of work explores her childhood and family relationships in bright, layered paintings that I hadn't stopped thinking about since I saw them online. After visiting my gallery, we exchanged a couple of emails and agreed to try to find a time to meet again. Then she sent me a longer email that was so powerful, so moving, that it made me audibly exhale, take a moment, and then reread. "Sarah, I actually just might as well put my cards on the table," she wrote, explaining that she'd never sought representation from a gallery before but felt compelled to reach out to me after our first, albeit brief, encounter. I loved that she wasn't afraid to be direct, to ask for what she wanted.

By the time I pulled into the parking lot, before I saw her work in person, I knew I was going to ask her to join SGG's roster, which I told her the moment I hugged her hello. Amy is in her sixties, has short blondish hair, and cool, thick-rimmed glasses. An artist's glasses. She was wearing a yellow sweater, jeans, and booties and introduced me to her husband, quick to praise him for his support of her artistic career.

The exhibition was huge—more than seventy pieces, some with accompanying poems, spread over two rooms—and as Amy explained each panel and the topics she was exploring, I began to feel as if I'd known her my whole life. There was something about the way words came out of her mouth, her gestures, and her sarcastic asides that felt so familiar. I thought about Mom, who also had short hair and was also a big fan of the sarcastic barb.

In front of one big series of portraits, Amy shared a story of childhood trauma that led her to become an artist. My eyes filled with tears as she explained the event that changed her, something she didn't share with anyone else until she was thirty-four and both of her parents had passed away. We hugged again; I apologized for crying and thanked her for feeling comfortable enough to share this part of her story. "I feel like I've known you forever," she said, and we both laughed as we continued to walk through the exhibition.

We agreed that Amy's first show at SGG would take place the next summer. Her work is exquisite, and I promised her I'd do everything in my power to make it a success from a sales perspective. I had to drive on to Cleveland after our meeting, but I couldn't wait to see her again and get to know her better. I'm not sure I believe in fate, but I do make room for something I call "special powers," and Amy and I both knew something profound happened in the museum that afternoon.

I got in my car and thought about Amy and how I just added another woman to the roster of women like Mom. Amy was a composite of Mom's qualities—the short hair, the sarcasm. But was that it? Did Amy really remind me of Mom? The similarities weren't as strong as the ones I'd noted in Christiane, Sharon, or Susanne, and in fact, I felt as if I was trying to force the connection. I let my mind wander, tried harder to see something I loved about Mom in her, and returned to the moment when Amy told me about her childhood, about how she paints to help make sense of her life. I thought about her poetry, her willingness to be direct with me, and how she doesn't take herself too seriously even if—especially if—the topic is actually a serious one.

My body reacted almost before my mind understood what was happening. I felt my skin buzz with a feeling that was exhilarating but also wildly uncomfortable, something I liked but didn't recognize. And when I tell you it hit me, it *hit* me. What I realized on Interstate

77 as I headed to Cleveland on a cold and rainy Saturday in October of 2023 was that this woman I suddenly felt a huge connection to and affection for wasn't like Mom at all.

The woman Amy reminded me of . . . was *me*. What the actual fuck?

You know how we have doppelgängers out there, and every once in a while, somebody will send you a photo of a person who looks like you? Or you see somebody you swear you've seen before and wonder how the world is so small? You're with me, right? These things happen. Except this . . . was not *that*. This moment was more like awareness cracking open after a long season of dormancy, the lifetime I'd spent hibernating in well-disguised self-loathing.

Thirty years or so of actively disliking everything about myself, plus ten years of therapy in which I learned to accept that there are likable qualities about me. Sounds absurd, I know, but the patterns are strong, and the patterns work really hard to make themselves known until you recognize them, address them, and conquer them. My pattern was hating myself, so the unwinding was bound to be slow and complicated. Don't believe me? Try it. Try saying something kind to yourself . . . about yourself. Right? Ew. Aside from megalomaniacs and people attending a self-help conference with a guru who's just walked across hot coals, I couldn't imagine who would ever do such a thing. I would look around on the street wondering if there were freaks of nature who actually *liked* themselves.

Starting at age forty, I crept toward a healthier perspective and started to get there five years into working with David. He finally helped me admit to myself—and say it aloud—that I liked myself. I still don't even want to type it because it feels fucking weird, and what happened on Interstate 77 took a long-ass time to achieve. I was driving north, the green highway signs telling me where to exit, what city I was approaching next. I imagined what it would look like if the signs correlated with the new order of things, the payoff for pulling myself out of the pain I'd disguised for so long under a thick armor of achievement.

FRIENDSHIP. Right there at exit 16.

THERAPY. Exit 19.

LOVE. Exit 22.

ART GALLERY. Exit 24.

The signs were all there for me, available to me all along, but I hadn't known how to navigate them—I didn't believe in myself enough to choose these routes until I was forty. Until I was ready. Until I did the work. Until I believed I was worthy. Argh. This driving analogy isn't working as well as I'd like, but I want you to see what happened to me that day. I want you to know how it felt in my body, even if I looked manic to drivers in the passing lane, what with bursts of crying interrupted by head shaking and heavy bouts of mouth-open laughter.

I felt like I understood something about myself, as if I'd gotten a new glimpse of who I am. I finally saw myself in this life I've discovered and created, and the feeling in my body was something I still hesitate to name, except that I need to, because I'm a writer, for fuck's sake.

The feeling in my body was, and is, joy.

At SGG we say that art is joy. I now see what I was seeking. And if I started this quirky little memoir over again, perhaps I'd thread the concept of joy through the story more, making it part of the pesky *through line* writing teachers talk about. I might even change the title to *Chasing Joy*.

But I'm not starting over, because that's not the order of things for me. I'm just going to sit here, in the joy of this second ending.

ADDENDUM 1—PRETTY STUFF

My neighbor was the first person who told me I wasn't pretty.

Theresa didn't mean it to be cruel; she just made a matter-of-fact observation. She was sixteen and one of the three McLoughlin sisters who were our closest neighbors up the road. Bill and Brad were the older brothers—you've met them. I'd spend countless hours watching the sisters apply colorful drugstore makeup from shiny containers in acrylic trays that they stored in a small bedroom closet, transforming themselves into exotic beings who fit better on movie screens than on our rural hayfield farms.

My friend Diane and I were enthralled by Theresa. In our eleven-year-old minds, her age and experience made her an authority figure on just about everything. The three of us were sitting on the twin beds in my room at the farm, talking about what we might like to do when we grow up. I remember thinking that becoming a large-animal vet was a good idea, but Theresa thought we should consider becoming actresses or perhaps models. After contemplating a little more, her forefinger and thumb cupping her chin as she studied us both, she commented, "Sarah, you might have the figure to be a model one day, but Diane is the one who is pretty enough." That was the first time I realized I wasn't one of the beautiful girls.

When I was in the eighth grade, an entire group of boys reinforced what Theresa had suggested years before. We were in Mr. Ferris's advanced English class. His wife was the teacher who double-knotted my laces in kindergarten, before kids were so mean. The bell rang, we all took our seats, and then I saw what everyone else saw. On the chalkboard at the front of the room, somebody had drawn a huge picture of me with words and arrows to indicate certain flaws. One arrow pointed to my pale legs, chalked in solid white. Another pointed to my flat chest, where the artist or artists spelled out *FLAT* like a T-shirt decal. One more arrow pointed to the gap between my front teeth. And next to the picture, somebody had written *UGLY*. I sat in the back row. I remember thinking the worst part of the whole situation was that because I was in the back row, everybody in class could simply turn around to see how very true the drawing was—to confirm that I was ugly. Somehow, I thought that if only I had been sitting in the front row, they would see only the back of my head and not my ugly face, which burned hot with stifled tears and that special shame reserved for girls who feel like they'll never be enough. Mr. Ferris quickly erased the caricature, but I could still draw it today, every chalk stroke a permanent laceration on my memory.

Much later, when I was twenty-six, Mom and I attended an engagement brunch for one of the college besties, Nancy, who you've also met. We all ended up in one of those conversations about our looks, what we liked, and what we might want to change one day, if we could. Mom suggested that some of my friends, like Nancy and Missy, were beautiful girls, while others like *me* were simply attractive in our own, distinct ways. For real. She said this to me, in front of my best friends.

"But your looks aren't what matters," she claimed. "Who you are as a person is on the inside, and that's what counts."

"MOM!" I yelled at her. "Are you kidding me?"

At the time, I laughed instead of crying because I knew Mom didn't mean to be cruel. I knew her well enough to understand that she actually meant what all of the mom guides say, but I just wanted a mom who thought I was beautiful. I'd never told her the story about my neighbor or the boys from eighth grade because I didn't want to pass along my pain.

Fast-forward to 2020. I was getting closer to fifty, and I'd started a new cycle of worrying about wrinkles and the age spots that I keep calling freckles. I was simultaneously growing weary of worrying about how I look and decided to try to solve the problem with art. Yay for art . . . art is joy . . . everyone, buy more art!

A local artist named Joey Monsoon paints incredible portraits that make you hesitate when you first see them. Are they beautiful? Slightly grotesque? There are lots of floating ears, and even when he paints a real person, the portrait is clearly of them, but also . . . not them. "The thread that runs throughout my work is that people are imperfect," Joey says of his subjects. "They are people who have endured real life, and that living of a life has left marks on them on the exterior and interior." Hot damn, he gets it. Joey's very cool, trust me. I decided to ask him to paint a portrait of me, knowing that it would not make me look beautiful and instead would make me look complicated, like a version of me. I declared to myself that once the painting was complete, I would stop caring about what I look like, embrace my age, and no longer cringe at the fine lines, "freckles," and Droopy-Dog-ness of my cheeks. I would use art to inspire a change in perspective. Hurrah!

Guess what? Guess fucking what? The great conversion-via-art strategy didn't work! Not at all, not even for one day. I sometimes still emit an audible sigh when I see my aging face, and I too often succumb to the latest miracle serums served up by social media. That's okay. Because even though I'm not fully embracing the face-sliding phenomenon, on most days I like the way I look. Pretty or not, my face is my face, and I'm living a life that leaves marks.

ADDENDUM 2—THIS IS NOT A COOKBOOK

I can't tell you the whole story of getting fired, because, well, we all love Martha, don't we? We do. You just need to know that after she fired me and before I landed the next big job, I did certain things. I drank a whole bunch of martinis at the Red Cat around the corner from my apartment in Chelsea. I did a whole bunch of Barre Method classes because if I was going to be unemployed, I was going to look good. And I made a whole bunch of chocolate chip cookies in my quest to perfect them. Thirty-eight different batches, in fact. A tweak here, a tweak there. And then, the sea salt.

MARTHA-STEWART-FIRED-ME COOKIES

Ingredients

- 2 sticks salted butter, softened
- ½ cup granulated sugar
- 1 cup packed dark brown sugar
- ½ cup packed light brown sugar
- 2 large eggs, room temperature

- 2 tsp. vanilla extract
- 2¾ cups (12 oz.) all-purpose flour
- ¼ tsp. smallish-to-medium-grain sea salt for batter, more for topping
- 1 tsp. baking soda
- 1½ tsp. baking powder
- 2¼ cups semisweet chocolate chips or chunks (chunks are better, chopped up a bit for texture, but you should use one and a half 16-ounce bags—definitely more than typically called for)

Instructions

1. Preheat oven to 360 degrees. Cream butter, sugar, and brown sugar until the mixture is nice and fluffy (approximately 3 minutes on medium-high speed—this seems like forever, so watch the clock and keep at it).
2. Add both eggs and the vanilla and beat for an additional 2 minutes (again, this feels like a long time).
3. Add baking soda, baking powder, a bit of salt, and flour until cookie batter is fully incorporated. Finally, add chocolate pieces and mix until well distributed.
4. Chill dough for 14–36 hours if you want them to be the best cookies ever. If you cannot chill the dough, they will still be amazing, I promise!
5. The cookie batter will be somewhat thick and quite sticky, so use your hands to plop balls of dough onto a baking sheet lined with parchment paper. I prefer dough balls slightly larger than a quarter (8 per sheet), but make whatever size you like; just be sure to adjust the baking time accordingly.
6. Sprinkle some sea salt over them before they go in the oven.
7. Bake for 10 minutes, until the edges are golden brown but the center is still light.

8. Remove from heat, slam down to flatten out a bit (okay, so I stole this from another recipe that is super popular; it helps keep them chewy in the middle), do another sprinkle of sea salt, and allow the cookies to stay on the cookie sheet for an additional 2 minutes.
9. Transfer cookies to a room-temperature, nonporous surface to cool for at least 3–5 minutes before serving.
10. You can reuse the parchment; just brush off the excess salt.

ACKNOWLEDGMENTS

I'm a Gormley all the way. Except for the healthy dose of Cameron. I adore my complicated, fucked-up family, and the genetic part of my Venn diagram is strong. Jane and Joe didn't have a choice about getting a little sister. I'm stunned that they still like me, especially after I tattled when they ran off to play and left me behind with the babysitter, who later spanked them and sent them to bed early. People don't always think we look alike, but when we're next to each other, we look like we belong together. Thank you, Jane and Joe, for no longer calling me "Ramona" and being nice to me even when you kind of want to punch me in the face.

Salt Creek Farm raised me. The hills and the woods and the caves and the barns and the church and the pond and the bridges and the fields dotted with black cows and Salt Creek itself. Before I knew anything different existed, I knew I was lucky to wake up in that house, on that land, and feel the breeze coming through the screen of the big window near the foot of my bed. The gratitude I feel for growing up in that place is spiritual, like a hymn I'll never stop humming, like a prayer written just for me.

Unconditional love was not a concept I understood well and one I still struggle with sometimes. But there's a group of gals I met at DePauw University who seemingly have been put into my life to force me to appreciate that such a thing exists. I call them "the girls" and call them—and call upon them—every day. Brooks, Fran, Gingy, Hegman, Madalyn, Nancy, Niner, Shawna, Tippett, and Tucker: I cannot fathom where or who I would be today without the force of you. I wrote an essay that was rejected by Modern Love about how much I feel you are a part of me, as if I carry you all in my body when I move through the day. Whether you know it or not, you've been carrying me all of this time, too.

Tippett, Hegman, and Nancy have also been a constant part of the reading, reviewing, and editing team, and they've acted interested all along, even if they were faking. I'm fairly needy. Tippett requested a special shout-out for removing thirty-seven fucks from the final manuscript. Thank you, Tippett, and also, fuck you. I love you and your Tiny Clay Books.

The Order of Things would not exist without Ruthie Ackerman telling me to "go deeper" and to "show instead of tell" during a full year of her classes as I worked on and finished the first draft. The next year, there was a retreat, a new outline, manuscript revisions, and quick check-ins. Ruthie, the rigor of your deadlines and the class structure helped me in ways I appreciate more every day. Thank you for your patience and support and for offering to read my essays aloud because I always start crying. Your immense talent is matched by your huge heart, and I'm so lucky to know you.

Christie Tate, you know how much I love to call you a *New York Times* bestselling author as loud as I can to embarrass you in public. Yes, you are a big deal. But you're also one of the funniest, snarkiest, grooviest people I've ever known. Even when I forced my way into your orbit for book stuff, I didn't have any idea how much knowledge you would impart to me as a writer and as a human being. I'm hoping that if I keep paying you for editing help, you'll keep being my friend.

Before the I'm-going-to-write-a-book writing teachers, I had other teachers, the people who shaped me and made me fall in love with the written word: Linda Bates at Chandlersville Elementary, Dean Harper at Duncan Falls Junior High, Janeen Lepp at Philo High School, and Wayne Glausser at DePauw University. Mrs. Bates taught us how to "get lost" in reading; Dean Harper helped me publish a poem about a pencil sharpener in a literary magazine; Dr.

Lepp pushed me to read critically and write with precision, her red pen always at the ready to catch errors and suggest a rewrite; Wayne took me on as an advisee during my freshman year when things were pretty rough for me. He stuck with me through my thesis on Raymond Carver and never complained (at least to me) about my neurotic paralysis and months of self-doubt. My dream book club would include these gorgeous people, and the fact that a little girl from Chandlersville, Ohio, was lucky enough to be exposed to their brilliance isn't lost on me.

Before the art gallery, there was corporate work, with many bosses over many years. Some terrible bosses, some okay bosses, and one exceptional boss. Rich Gelfond truly believed in me, taught me, guided my career, and basically adopted me—even though I had a penchant for pissing him off. A fellow therapy head, Rich knew what modulation was long before I did and repeatedly told me that "things are never as bad as they look or as good as they seem." He also lets me stay at his gorgeous estate in Southampton, but that's not why I love him. Not at all.

Therapist David. There should be an Oscars-style event for therapists where we get to publicly praise these saviors. He helped me change my life. He changed my life. Period. I've known David more than ten years and have paid him so much money, it's a good fucking thing it's all working out. I want to reverse roles just once and say, "Let's go slowly, David. Why don't you try to tell me how much you've helped change Sarah's life? Is it hard for you to take credit for what you've done for her? Why do you think that is?" Nothing feels better than making David laugh, and I'm so thankful I found him when I needed him most. David, your blue suit is probably still too big, but now that we only talk on the phone, I don't have to think about such things. Thank you for leading me to this version of life. I wouldn't be who I am today without you.

Camillus Musselman. All of the syllables of you. I hope I never tire of saying your name or hearing you say mine. Thank you for supporting me so relentlessly. For putting up with me when I'm hungry and when I lose my keys/phone/wallet and when I don't close lids properly. Thank you for making me breakfast sandwiches. Thank you for coming to pick me up that morning back in 2017. Thank you for liking me and loving me, and thank you most of all for letting me love you. Being good at loving you is the best gold star of all.

ABOUT THE AUTHOR

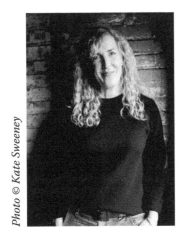

Photo © Kate Sweeney

Sarah Gormley is a writer and art gallery owner living in Columbus, Ohio. Her undergraduate degree from DePauw University reinforced an early love for literature and writing, while the heavy sprinkling of liberal-arts fairy dust taught her how to analyze and articulate a clear point of view. She rounded out this foundation with concentrations in marketing and operations from the University of Chicago Graduate School of Business.

Her marketing career included work with several global brands, including IMAX, Martha Stewart, Girl Scouts of the USA, and Adobe. Gormley was honored as one of 2015's Forty Women to Watch over 40, and she has been featured in *Forbes* and the CMO Club. In June 2019, she was invited to deliver the class address at her DePauw University class reunion and regrets not having her hair blown out.

Today, Gormley owns a contemporary art gallery, Sarah Gormley Gallery (SGG), in downtown Columbus, Ohio. The gallery operates based on the belief that original art can be a source of joy for everyone and actively eschews pretense of any kind. She opened the gallery in 2019, twenty-five years after her Grandma Cameron gifted her with her first piece of art.

Printed in the USA
CPSIA information can be obtained
at www.ICGtesting.com
CBHW021802190824
13420CB00001B/2